THE
DUBROW
KETO
FUSION
DIET

THE
DUBROW
KETO
FUSION
DIET

THE ULTIMATE PLAN FOR INTERVAL EATING
AND SUSTAINABLE FAT BURNING

HEATHER DUBROW AND TERRY DUBROW, M.D., F.A.C.S.

WM

WILLIAM MORROW

An Imprint of HarperCollins*Publishers*

This book is written as a source of information about the keto diet and intermittent fasting. It is based on the research and observations of the authors, one of whom is a medical doctor. The information contained in this book should by no means be considered a substitute for the advice of a qualified medical professional, who should always be consulted before beginning any diet, exercise, or other health program.

The information in this book has been carefully researched, and all efforts have been made to ensure accuracy as of the date published. Readers, particularly those with existing health problems and those who take prescription medications, are cautioned to consult with a health professional about specific recommendations for supplements, and the appropriate dosages. The author and the publisher expressly disclaim responsibility for any adverse effects arising from the use or application of the information contained in this book.

Quotes included throughout attributed to individuals were gathered from early testers of the Dubrow Keto Fusion Diet.

THE DUBROW KETO FUSION DIET. Copyright © 2020 by Frontal Lobe Productions, Inc. All rights reserved. Printed in the United States of America. No part of this book may be used or reproduced in any manner whatsoever without written permission except in the case of brief quotations embodied in critical articles and reviews. For information, address HarperCollins Publishers, 195 Broadway, New York, NY 10007.

HarperCollins books may be purchased for educational, business, or sales promotional use. For information, please email the Special Markets Department at SPsales@harpercollins.com.

FIRST EDITION

Library of Congress Cataloging-in-Publication Data has been applied for.

ISBN 978-0-06-298432-6

20 21 22 23 24   LSC   10 9 8 7 6 5 4 3 2 1

I dedicate this book to my amazing, larger-than-life husband! I knew if we kept pushing, we could find a way to stay fit and healthy, and still have onion rings now and again! After almost a quarter of a century as partners, I love that we continue to learn and grow together—and still laugh along the way! I love you, Honyi!

I dedicate this book to my two favorite things in this world (not including my kids): my wife and science. To my wife, who has taught me how to strive to live the healthiest, happiest, and longest life I possibly can so that I can enjoy and inspire my kids and my patients to do the same. And to science; how else could we devise an easy-to-follow, stress-free way to eat healthfully without starving ourselves . . . and to enjoy the foods we all know are crucial to living strong, healthy lives? Cheers!

CONTENTS

CONTENTS

viii

FOREWORD

I rarely get excited about books dedicated to diet and exercise. But I found myself truly becoming excited as I read the Dubrows' book. Finally, a series of evidence-based recommendations about diet with straightforward recommendations for exercises that anyone can follow and from which they can optimally benefit.

From the outset, I could tell the Keto Fusion plan was something from which I could personally benefit. As someone who has metabolic syndrome and is therefore acutely aware of the importance of addressing insulin resistance, I have been making efforts to stay on a ketogenic diet. I am convinced that for patients like myself, insulin is a much more important story than most people know (this hunch is validated by Dr. Dubrow in the pages ahead). Addressing our dependence on carbohydrates and eliminating them from our diet must become a priority. But staying on a diet with extreme carbohydrate restriction can be challenging; I can tell you firsthand.

Of late, I have noticed myself haphazardly liberalizing my diet, and I have been concerned that I may be sliding into problematic territory. Now with the guidance of the "fusion" of evidenced-based nutritional recommendations created by the Dubrows, I have a sensible structure to get back on track. With the use of fasting, increased intake of certain types of fats, and low glycemic-index carbohydrates, I can see how applying this trio of ideas to create a road forward will give me the ability to maintain indefinitely and achieve my dietary goals.

The Dubrow Keto Fusion Diet makes currently available wisdom on our diets understandable and the recommendations are something that anyone should be able to follow. Here are a few standouts:

* The science is here, it is accurate, and it is interpreted in a manner that anyone can understand.
* The exercise element is sensible and will provide a framework that will benefit all.
* Heather's voice is funny, fresh, and, most important I think, she's honest in a way that takes the sting out of certain dieting realities.
* And, one last, maybe favorite element: There are considerations for those of us (me and Dr. Dubrow at least . . . I'm pretty sure Heather is actually ageless) who have found ourselves facing the inevitable consequences of being a biological being, namely aging.

I know every review of a wellness book extolls the virtues and suggests you put away everything that has come before. But that is truly the case here: *Put away everything else.* This is the state of the art reviewed by a knowledgeable clinician who interprets the buzz and confusion out there.

It's all here. Even recommendations for the basic maintenance of our mental health. Congratulations to the Dubrows for creating a program that will make a difference in your health and well-being.

Dr. Drew Pinsky

THE
DUBROW
KETO
FUSION
DIET

INTRODUCTION

Let us start by saying *thank you* for picking up this book.

We are thrilled to share our second diet book with you! When *The Dubrow Diet* came out in October 2018, we were blown away by the response and the results. We heard from so many readers who reached out on social media or called in during our podcasts, *Heather Dubrow's World* and *Dr. and Mrs. Guinea Pig*. We even got to do in-person interviews with some of our most successful Dubrow dieters, which was truly an honor and left us seriously impressed.

Publishing a book was one of the most impactful ways we've ever connected with people who've followed us through our time in the reality TV spotlight. (It was also great to connect with those three people who picked up the book without a clue about who we were and just wanted to lose weight. Just kidding about the three people; maybe there were ten?) The knowledge that people were using our diet to change their bodies and lives, no matter how they came to find the book, was inspiring and awesome.

Now, you might be wondering, "Why do it again?"

There are a few reasons. The first is that it's fun. Sure, writing a book is time-consuming and hard work, but there's something so cool about creating an actual thing that's going to get picked up at a bookstore or downloaded onto an e-reader or smartphone or, who knows, even a watch. The second is that for as solid as the Dubrow Diet was (and still is), there were some people who experienced a little more hunger than they liked, and they felt this was a deterrent to sticking with the diet long-term. The third reason is Steve from Google. No last name. Just Steve. We'll explain.

Steve from Google

Early in 2019, we got an email that said simply, "This is Steve from Google. We wanted to let you know that 'Dubrow diet' was the second most searched term in the diet category for all of 2018." Our first response was, OK, *Steve* . . . this is obviously a scam just trying to get us to spend money. But after looking into it, we found out that it was legitimate—even though our book didn't come out until October of 2018, the interest was so high that we somehow landed near the top of the search list for the year. Crazy!

So, our second response was—if we were #2, what was #1? The keto diet. That's what took the top spot. Hmm. Dubrow diet and keto, we wondered, is it possible that the two belong together?

As we began contemplating this fusion, we also heard from some of the Dubrow dieters that they were pulling in keto elements and creating their own hybrid. Okay, we thought, it's possible that they are really on to something.

Confessions of One-Time Keto Doubters

Now, obviously Steve's email wasn't the first time we had heard about keto. In fact, this leads to a confession that we should just get out of the way early on. We *might* have said some things about the keto diet in the past that we regret. Things like this:

"I think the keto diet—no offense to those who like it— physiologically ... as a doctor ... it's really dumb." —*Terry Dubrow, M.D.*

"In practical terms, I don't like the keto diet. It's not sustainable and the thing about the keto diet is, the minute you cheat, it's over, you're out of that ketonic state and any result you had is absolutely gone." —*Heather Dubrow*

Yes, yes ... those statements were made by the very same Dubrows who sit here writing to you today, introducing their new diet book that is based *in part* (that's a key phrase here) on the keto diet. To be fair, we had been hearing from a lot of friends who were following the keto diet, and they were pretty miserable. Most of them just couldn't tolerate the very high fat requirements of the diet for more than a couple of days.

Yet it was obvious that there was an undeniable draw to keto and its promised results. We—well, Terry especially because he always likes to do things in his own "Terry-ish" way—wondered if this type of diet had to be done the conventional way.

Or could it be made better?

He can relate what happened when he started searching for answers to this question.

Falling for Keto

I have to admit that calling something "dumb" when you don't know a lot about it is kind of . . . not so smart. But here's the thing about M.D.s—we can sometimes be a little shortsighted. We often exist in such a bubble, especially specialty surgeons like myself, that when we emerge, we try to do rapid-fire consumption of information on a lot of different topics. And this can lead to a dissemination of opinions that are less than fully considered. This was my initial experience with the ketogenic diet.

My subsequent experiences involved more in-depth personal exploration on the topic. I started reading about the history of the ketogenic diet and how it was first developed and used in the 1920s as a treatment for epilepsy. I read about how it was designed to mimic fasting, the metabolic effects of which I love. The world's introduction to the keto diet remained, for decades, mostly limited to the clinical settings as a treatment for epilepsy. However, use of the diet fell significantly once alternative pharmaceutical approaches became available.

The diet came back into favor after *Dateline* aired a remarkable story in 1994 featuring a young boy named Charlie Abrahams who had been diagnosed with epilepsy and was experiencing unrelenting seizures that couldn't be resolved by medications, surgery, or any other type of approach. Feeling desperate, Charlie's father, Jim, began his own search for answers and unearthed the 1920s research on the ketogenic diet—the very same diet that had been used successfully before, but had never been mentioned to the Abrahams family as a potential solution.

They sought out the team at Johns Hopkins University who had originally introduced the ketogenic diet, and with their help, put Charlie on the diet. "His seizures started to diminish almost immediately," recalled Jim Abrahams in the *Dateline* special. One month of strict adherence to the ketogenic diet eliminated them entirely.

As a parent, I can only imagine the profound relief this produced. As a doctor, I marvel at the ways that forward progress can sometimes require looking back. After all, it was over two thousand years ago that the famous Greek physician Hippocrates supposedly said, "Let food be thy medicine." But like I mentioned, doctors can be shortsighted. . . .

Needless to say, I was intrigued by the awesome power of the ketogenic diet, which works by shifting the body to utilize ketones, which are generated from dietary fats or stored body fat, instead of glucose, generated from carbohydrates or stored carbs (in the form of glycogen), for energy. Ketones have proven to have neuroprotective effects, perhaps because they seem to reduce inflammation in the brain and encourage the growth of new neurons. Researchers continue to explore exactly why ketones are so beneficial to brain health, and how it is they help improve metabolic disorders such as type 2 diabetes, as well as diseases like epilepsy and Alzheimer's.

The original—or classic—ketogenic diet used to cure and treat disease allows only 4 percent carbs and requires your dietary intake to consist of 90 percent fat. In case you can't tell, that is *a lot* of fat, and eating this much fat often requires eating tons of meat and eggs—not to mention slugging down oils all day long. In clinical settings, it's considered essential to meet this 90-percent fat requirement and there's 0-percent flexibility for falling off track. The consequences can be serious: halted healing and a return of symptoms.

When it comes to weight loss, a lot of keto proponents insist that this same seriousness is required for results. But no one who is following a diet to produce weight loss can commit to a diet made up of 90, or even 80, percent fat—no matter how motivated you think you are, the prospect of weight loss is not enough to justify eating such an unpalatable amount of fat each day.

Which is why it's so exciting that there has been a big push over the last few decades to find "keto-ish" ways of eating that relax the fat requirements some and increase the carbohydrate intake. When I started reading the research on these options, I found a favorite called the low-glycemic index treatment (LGIT) diet, which was defined as "liberalized keto"—that is, keto that's been freed from extreme restrictions. Of the various types now being used in clinical settings, this was the one that seemed to me to be the most sustainable, because it allowed more than double the amount of carbohydrates found in most ketogenic diets.

If you have ever tried to follow a keto diet before, you understand how significant this is. The extreme low carbs required by most keto diets can lead to headache, constipation, nausea, fatigue, bad breath, leg cramps. . . . It's a lot to endure for the sake of weight loss. I knew that this smarter carb consumption was going to have a central role in the next evolution of how the Dubrows would eat.

Creating the Fusion

When Heather and I created the Dubrow Diet, the program was in large part a response to the constant requests we would get about how we keep ourselves in shape. We were surprised by how much fun it was to distill our at-home diet into one that we could share with others. I knew there were some people who didn't enjoy the longer fasting requirement (sixteen hours is a long time!) and felt that this kept them from sticking to it long-term. And this is why I knew our diet could get better. Sometimes you need other people to point out where improvements can be made, because you can't see those gaps for yourself.

In a way, the information we received from Steve from Google was the first lightbulb: maybe there's room for keto somewhere? But I knew it would be tough to shake my early opinions on the diet, which were formed after watching Heather's assistant struggle to ingest tablespoons of straight oil. Again: not sustainable (unless you are trying to eliminate seizures).

The answer revealed itself through a little bit of diet design creativity. We knew three things:

1. We wanted to retain the practice of intermittent fasting, which is so essential to resetting cellular metabolism and has benefits that should not be missed in disease prevention and longevity.
2. Keto could be tolerated part-time, and nutritional ketosis could help extend the benefits of fasting.
3. Low-glycemic carbs could be included as a way to minimize the unpleasant side effects of classic keto.

When we put these three dietary details together, the Dubrow Keto Fusion Diet (DKFD) came to be. By combining these dietary approaches, the DKFD initiates a metabolic reconstruction that will help you burn stored fat, eliminate the cellular detritus that so often sparks disease and accelerates aging, feel sharper mentally, experience an increase in energy . . . and more.

We cannot wait for you to try it.

The Future of the Ketogenic Diet

In the DKFD, we've borrowed from the classic ketogenic diet to create an approach to eating that will help you achieve weight loss (along with the benefits listed above). While researching and refining our diet, we learned that this original keto has origins that should not be forgotten, and a power to heal and help those in great need. We encourage you to explore some of this history, and to evaluate the clinical use of the ketogenic diet in its many forms if you or someone you love is affected by epilepsy, type 2 diabetes, or Alzheimer's disease and other neurologic disorders. You never know if a dietary approach may produce some relief, or even eliminate symptoms as it did for Charlie Abrahams. You can read more about Charlie's story on the Charlie Foundation's website.

Take the 5% Pledge—A Modest Goal with Major Payoff

Contemplating your weight loss goal at the start of a diet can feel a lot like staring up at Mount Everest—it seems like an *impossible* climb. After years of frustrating experiences with dieting, we know exactly how daunting it is. That's why the DKFD encourages a different approach: We want you to take what we call The 5% Pledge.

The 5% Pledge is our research-backed recommendation to aim to lose just 5 percent of your current weight. If you weigh 160 pounds, this would be a goal to drop 8 pounds; at 185, you have just over 9 pounds to lose . . . 200 pounds, you're looking at a goal of 10 pounds.

A lot of people say they want to lose 20 to 40 pounds, but for most that trek is too long and they often get discouraged and fall off track. Research shows that just a 5-percent weight loss can have major health benefits, including improving:

* Insulin sensitivity.
* Risk factors for heart disease, e.g., blood pressure and triglyceride concentration.
* Overall metabolic function.

We encourage you to start with a 5-percent goal. You can do it! #IPledgeDKFD

Even though we are writing this book together, we would read it very differently—Terry would dive into the science and want to understand the "why" behind every little thing (I mean, to an annoying degree). Heather (that's me), would skim for some science-y words that would make me feel that it was legitimate, and then probably jump to the actual diet. My philosophy: *Just cut to the chase and tell me what to eat!*

You can use this book according to what type of reader you are, whether you're a Heather or a Terry (or a fusion of the two!). If you are more like Terry, you will probably want to read the first three chapters in full, as these were written mostly by him and are therefore chock-full of the metabolic science that supports the Dubrow Keto Fusion Diet.

If you are more like *moi*, you could jump to Part II of the book, where you will find the food lists for shopping, snacks, and meals, and the DKFD recipes. You'll also find super-fun photos of our family in our favorite place in the house: our kitchen. I pretty much hijacked this latter part of the book because it's way more fun (sorry, Terry).

Basically, this book is like a mullet: business in the front and party in the back.

So there you go: You can now make an informed decision about where you want to start with the book. If you're a Heather/Terry hybrid, feel free to jump around however you like. But don't say I didn't warn you about the brainiac stuff you'll find in the beginning.

No matter how you want to ingest the material, we promise it's easier than ingesting pure oil, and we're sure you'll love the results. Be sure to watch out for the quotes sprinkled throughout the book—these were gathered from early testers of the diet, and they shared with us what they loved! We can't wait for you to try the DKFD out in your own life!

PART I

The Science of the DKFD

CHAPTER 1

BEHIND THE SCENES OF A METABOLIC MELTDOWN (AND HOW YOU CAN RECOVER)

You probably don't spend a lot of time scrolling through the websites of the Centers for Disease Control and Prevention or the World Health Organization, but if you did, you'd find some stats that are scarier than any episode of *Stranger Things*. I'm talking about some seriously frightening stuff. Here's some of the information I've seen:

* Over 70 percent of Americans are either overweight or obese.
* Worldwide obesity has nearly tripled since 1975.
* Most of the world's population live in countries where overweight and obesity kills more people than underweight.
* Obesity-related conditions include heart disease, stroke, type 2 diabetes, and certain types of cancer, which are some of the leading causes of preventable, premature death.
* Obesity is preventable.

At a time when medical advances are so incredible that they seem sprung straight out of science fiction, these facts are almost impossible to believe, yet they are not the stuff of make-believe. We appear to be in the midst of a full-blown metabolic meltdown.

The obesity epidemic has been a decades-long development, but in our own bodies, it can feel as though significant change happens overnight—we look away from the mirror for one minute and return to find a muffin top or man boobs. I'll tell you a little story as an example.

In June of 2019, my lovely wife, Heather, and I went to France for a two-week vacation. As one of the busiest plastic surgeons in the world, taking a vacation this long is not something I can do regularly; I have patients depending on me and a full staff of twenty-three who rely on me to keep them busy and employed. But between my medical practice and shooting episodes of *Botched* and *License to Kill*, I had been working nonstop for several months. I like to work—love it, actually—but I needed a break. Off to France we went.

Once we arrived, we proceeded to eat whatever we wanted. I'm talking pizza, bread, croissants, cheese, and then more bread, in outrageous excess—and whatever we ate, we drank twice that. For two weeks, it was all high-carb, high-fat, high-alcohol, and minimal exercise.

Fans of our podcast or shows know that this is the opposite of our normal routine (except for the fat part). At home in Newport Beach, California, we eat very low-carb, fill up on plenty of high-quality fats, and . . . well, the drinking part isn't that different . . . but we both exercise diligently and daily.

What would you think the consequences—or let's call it the metabolic price—of this time in France might be? I can't speak for Heather because she was very coy about her stats after this trip, but for me, the price I paid was 14 pounds. I *gained* 14 pounds in two weeks. That's a pound a day. My pants were tight, my shirts hugged my body in a way that I hate, my usual baseline high energy level was completely sapped. I was blown away by how awful I felt—and frankly, how quickly it happened.

Now, my experience was at an accelerated rate (maybe it's the European conversion rate?), but I think for a lot of people this is how weight gain happens—you make a seemingly innocuous choice once, or twice, and don't realize that the result is that your body makes a metabolic preference for fat storage. Since you likely aren't aware this is happening, you don't go after this extra baggage right away, and it settles in. Once it's comfortable, it even starts to invite additional fatty tissue to join the party. And of course the longer it's there, the more stubborn this baggage seems to become.

Luckily for me, I knew how to correct my metabolism in a way that would return my physique to its prior form. A couple of years ago, my biohacking approach would have relied primarily upon the practice of intermittent fasting as *the* metabolic solution. This practice, which Heather and I refer to as interval eating, is at the core of our previous book, *The Dubrow Diet*. But we've gotten smarter, and our strategies have gotten better and—this is key—more sustainable.

Don't get me wrong—fasting is fantastic, and it's still one of the primary practices in the Dubrow Keto Fusion Diet (DKFD), but we've identified a superior way to restore metabolic function to its optimal state. This method includes fasting at a shortened duration, that is, fewer hours of feeling hungry, combined with a ketogenic-based eating strategy that essentially acts as a fast extender.

What I've discovered is that this is the most civilized, sensible, no-suffering-required way to reset and restore your internal biology related to weight and metabolism. So while I panicked at the weight gain, that didn't last long, because, being me, I shifted my focus to fixing the problem. I turned to this powerful fusion strategy to drop what I started referring to as my "France 14," and it was indeed the perfect fix, helping me return to my normal weight within twenty-one days.

With that endorsement, you may be eager to get to know the DKFD better, and soon enough you will. However, before we get into the specifics of the diet, I want to first address the most common factors behind the unprecedented weight gain affecting millions in this country, and billions across the globe.

The Trouble with the Way We Eat Today

A lot of people have gained a lot of weight over the last several decades. There's a lot of theorizing about why this has happened, and by theorizing, I mean that people like to talk nonstop about the origins of obesity. Since I'm about to do exactly that, I won't be too critical of these efforts at explanation, but I will say this: As someone who's more interested in solutions, I'm not going to make you read two hundred pages on the "why," because I want to get you to the "what can we do about it" section quickly. That said, a little bit of understanding is helpful and can strengthen the motivation needed to support a change in your health habits.

Looking back at our trip to France, I can isolate the three primary factors involved in weight gain:

1. Overreliance on carbohydrates.
2. Overnutrition.
3. Minimal exercise.

I mean, doesn't that already sound like the perfect recipe for vacation weight gain? The problem is that in most cases, these aren't vacation habits, but everyday ones. So while it's fairly easy to dial back on bad habits after indulging in them for a brief period, it's much more challenging to recalibrate your entire lifestyle to allow you to reach a healthy weight.

It must be pointed out that while there is some degree of personal responsibility here, there are large, systemic, even sneaky forces that have established an environment in which high-carb and high-calorie eating are the easiest (and seemingly least expensive) route for most people to take. And because we are, every single one of us, so crunched for time, squeezing exercise in is a constant challenge (see Chapter 8 for our favorite, most efficient workouts).

Let's look a little further at each of these factors and how they're programming people to get—and stay—fat.

1. Overreliance on Carbohydrates

Ahh, the carbohydrate. What's not to love? It's bready, chewy, sweet, sometimes crunchy . . . always satisfying in that distinctly carb-y way. Carbs seem to satiate a hunger pang faster than just about anything else. Think of it this way: If you're absolutely famished when you get home, and you run into your kitchen looking for relief, what do you grab? Do you reach for that half a steak you had left over from dinner the night before or do you grab the bag of chips on the counter and start plowing through them? Chips every single time.

Of course, there are different kinds of carbs, and what you choose to eat is significant. Vegetables, for example, are full of high-quality carbohydrates, also known as "fresh carbs."

But that's not what you grab when you run into the kitchen hungry. You go for what Heather and I call "factory carbs"—those highly processed foods made from refined flours and sugars, like breads, chips, cookies, pastas, pizza, etc.

There's an undeniable biological appeal to factory carbs: They are simple for your body to break down and use for energy (which is why in the panic of hunger, you know to reach for the chips). When you eat factory carbs, the raw materials are rapidly converted to blood sugar (glucose). As your blood sugar rises, your pancreas kicks out insulin so that your cells can use the fuel that's just come in.

Insulin: The Anti-Diet

Eating processed carbs triggers a sudden surge in blood sugar, and this surge then requires your body to respond by rapidly releasing insulin. Although you need insulin to move blood sugar into cells for use, big spikes of it can lead to sugar being converted to fat, and these big spikes prevent fat from being broken down . . . this is why I like to call insulin the anti-diet. Keep this in mind as we introduce more of the theory behind the DKFD, much of which revolves around eating to keep insulin low.

There's another reason, however, that these types of carbs are so appealing—they are *everywhere*. Plus, they're usually dressed up in pretty packaging with bright colors and maybe even a cute little cartoon character (to ensure that your kids want them so desperately that they'll throw a tantrum in the middle of a grocery store aisle until you relent). They are nearly impossible to avoid, and this is no accident. Not by a long shot.

The availability of factory carbs is intertwined with the demonization of fats found in foods, with the fat as bad guy coming first in the dietary timeline. In a 2008 research paper titled "How the Ideology of Low Fat Conquered America," Professor Ann F. La Berge of Virginia Tech discussed this timeline in detail. She noted a series of studies presented during the 1950s and '60s that suggested a possible connection between saturated fats and heart disease. This connection was referred to as the diet-heart hypothesis because it was just speculation that eating saturated fats raised serum cholesterol and then caused heart disease.

The fact that there wasn't proof to these claims didn't stop the public from taking them as fact, largely thanks to a government endorsement of the theory in 1977. It also didn't seem to matter that the studies that started it all had focused on people considered to have higher risk for developing heart disease; the "stay away from fats" decree was issued for all.

As the message grew increasingly louder, it changed the foods that were produced and sold, which in turn changed how people ate. Whole milk was pushed out in favor of nonfat milk; low-fat cheeses and yogurts were all the rage; low-fat cookies, tortillas, and cereals became the healthiest foods on the market. These foods were promoted as lower in fat and therefore lower in calories, and bingo: better for you.

The American Heart Association even came up with a sticker to slap onto many of these foods to let consumers know exactly how healthy they were. (If you were an adult or young adult in the early '90s, you probably remember these stickers that said "Heart Healthy." Did you know that companies paid to be able to use this official sign of approval? I'm going to guess no.) No one was immune to this propaganda; at least this doctor wasn't—I was crazy about carbs in my twenties and thirties, right around when they were being promoted as so good for you!

The major problem with all this was that fat brought flavor to foods, and something had to replace the tastiness that was lost. And this is where sugar, the first factory carb, comes in. All those low-fat and nonfat foods, now being promoted as heart healthy, were *loaded* with sugar. What no one really saw at the time was exactly how much sugar had to be added to recover the flavor and make food palatable. Hint—it was a lot.

Do "Low-Fat" Foods Have Fewer Calories?

When you compare a pure carbohydrate gram to one that's pure fat, the fat will have more calories; fat has 9 calories compared to carbohydrate's 4 (protein also has 4 calories per gram). But when we're talking about processed low-fat foods, the calorie difference is typically not much. This is because the amount of sugar needed to add flavor in the absence of fat is so significant that it can increase the number of calories quickly. There is a nutrition difference: Sugar is processed quickly, leaving you hungry again in a flash; and unless you're running a marathon, it will soon get stored in your fat cells. Dietary fats, on the other hand, are slow-burning, and the right kind can help cushion and lubricate cell membranes and nerves. More to come on calories on page 23.

It was generally accepted that sugar and processed carbs were the better option when it came to your health. But just because one thing is bad doesn't automatically mean that another is good. How did we know these fat alternatives were the safer bet and better for our health? Well, because scientists at Harvard said they were.

It turns out, if we look back to when the first rumblings about fat and heart disease originated, we find that for a time there was a debate about whether it was fats or carbohydrates that were bad for the heart. Research published on both sides of the issue was batted around, and the debate waged on until 1967, when three Harvard-backed researchers published a study called "Dietary Fats, Carbohydrates and Atherosclerotic Vascular Disease." (I know this may sound only slightly less scandalous than *50 Shades of Grey*, but there's a juicy tale in here—just you wait.) These Ivy League guys came in and essentially said, "We looked at all the stuff on sugar and all the stuff on fat, and we're going to call it—fat is the bad guy." Argument over.

Or at least it seemed like it was over. Fifty years later, a woman researching the sugar industry uncovered information that showed that these Harvard doctors, whose opinions shaped so much of the Western diet for decades, had been paid by the sugar industry to prove that fat—not sugar—was the foe. Whoa.

What this tells us is that all the shifts in dietary advice, the rise of the low-fat movement, and the powerful product marketing were in large part orchestrated by the sugar industry, which stood to lose so much if sugar took the majority of the blame and fat went on to flourish. This paved the way for not just sugar, but all processed carbs, to be seen in the public eye as positive instead of as something that's more complex when it's eaten and processed by the body.

Whether you realize it or not, this stubborn and complicated history has probably impacted how you view food today. Specifically, if you have an inexplicable fear of fat, it's likely a result of the low-fat/high-carb feud that started so many decades ago. A feud that spawned the popularity in low-fat diets, which have "helped fuel the twin epidemics of obesity and diabetes in America," as Dr. Dariush Mozaffarian of Tufts University wrote in 2015.

This heavy emphasis on carbs leads to a lot of internal trouble, specifically:

* Increased inflammation: As you eat a lot of carbs (like I used to . . . I was all about "carb loading" as an ex-endurance athlete) and avoid fats, what happens is a rapid peak rise in

blood glucose, which causes inflammation. If this inflammation is sustained, it can become chronic inflammation, which is a simmering, damaging sort of cellular heat that can injure cells, tissue, and DNA. This type of internal injury has been linked to type 2 diabetes, obesity, cancer, heart disease, and Alzheimer's.

* **Inhibition of fat burning:** Sudden surges in insulin lead to inhibition of lipolysis and inducement of lipogenesis and fat storage, as well as "carb cravings" due to the rapid peaks and troughs of blood glucose levels.

Let's Fix It: In the DKFD, you'll discover an approach to eating that will help undo the damage caused by a diet high in factory carbs. You will give your metabolism a break from the carb-initiated fat storage cycle and turn down the internal, disease-initiating fire of inflammation. This doesn't mean eliminating carbohydrates from your diet, but instead learning how and when to enjoy them.

The DKFD for Diabetics

If you have type 2 diabetes and you want to try this diet, the first line of business is to ask your personal physician if it's recommended. Since he or she will know your full health profile, they'll be able to speak to the safety of shifting to a keto-ish plus low-GI carb diet.

Generally speaking, research has shown that following this type of diet can lead to the need for less medication or even the cessation of meds in type 2 diabetics. The reason for this is the introduction of better glucose control via reduced glycemic response and improved insulin sensitivity.

If you are taking insulin, it will likely be important for you to monitor your morning insulin dose. In the Dubrow Keto Fusion Diet, the second window (the 8-hour Recharge) involves very low carbohydrates, so the regular morning insulin dose would have to potentially be lowered to account for a lower daytime blood glucose reading. At the beginning of the diet, careful glucose monitoring would be advised to prevent lowering the blood sugar values too far. Again, check with your personal doctor before beginning the diet.

2. Overnutrition

So, my time in the cafés of France revealed to me how too many carbs can set us up for weight gain; but too many calories can mean literal tummy trouble, too, especially if we're talking about an intake beyond your biological needs day after day.

The average American eats about 3,600 calories per day. If you are a farmer or construction worker or bicycle messenger, or you do anything that's physically demanding each day, this number might be right for you (in fact, you might need *more* calories). However, if you are sedentary the majority of the day—that is, you sit inside and stare at a computer for six to nine hours a day and then you go home and watch TV for three to four hours—this is way more than you need. If this is your lifestyle, you probably need closer to 1,500 to 2,200 calories.

Now, I like to think of us Dubrows as recovering calorie counters; both Heather and I spent years operating according to the "calories in/calories out" dogma, which says that if you burn more calories than you eat, you'll lose weight. In time, we both discovered that it wasn't a sustainable way to live nor is it chemically entirely accurate; and this is why neither the Dubrow Diet nor the DKFD require calorie counting. But, this sort of freedom isn't entirely free; you still need to pay attention to food quality and feelings of fullness.

In my experience, most people don't have any idea how many calories they eat each day. Research on eaters in England revealed that people may underestimate what they eat by as much as 50 percent; that means if you think you're eating 2,000 calories, you might actually be eating 3,000. That's a Whopper, well, actually almost a Double Whopper of a misread (a Double Whopper is about 950 calories).

Daily caloric excess does not come without consequences. The most obvious and well-known, of course, is weight gain, which is perhaps the least mysterious result of eating too many calories. It is merely an issue of supply and demand. Your body has specific nutrient demands, defined as your basal metabolic rate, and when you eat beyond these demands you supply more than what is needed. This oversupply gets stored in your cells (as fat) for later use.

Metabolic research reveals that there are additional types of internal dysfunction that can occur in response to overnutrition, some of which may set you up for further struggle with excess weight and the metabolic mayhem it can cause. Animal studies have shown that just three days of overeating can lead to hyperphagia—excessive hunger—and both insulin and leptin resistance. When your cells resist these two hormones, you are (1) at risk for developing type 2 diabetes and (2) likely to experience insatiable hunger and reduced caloric burn.

Eating too many calories each day is often a result of being disconnected from portions (portion distortion syndrome). For this reason, the DKFD Food Lists will provide you with foods and portion sizes. Use these portion sizes as a general suggestion of how much you'll want to eat of each food. If you follow the recipes in Chapter 6, these will already mostly adhere to these portion sizes.

Let's Fix It: As you shift your diet to be higher in quality fats and lower in processed carbohydrates, you will take advantage of biochemical signals in the body that can help control your appetite and make it easier to avoid the problem of overnutrition. Eating more dietary fats will help you feel fuller longer as they take longer than carbs and protein to digest.

We'll be talking more about the unique benefits of fat metabolism in Chapter 3.

3. Minimal Exercise

When you combine overnutrition with too little exercise, you put yourself on a one-way train to weight gain central. Exercise represents the only natural and healthy way to increase your body's utilization of calories. This means if you're going to consume more than your body needs, you better be prepared to bust your butt on the treadmill, today, tomorrow, and every day after that. Still, this is an imprecise solution—there's a gross unfairness about how much exercise it takes to burn a surprisingly small number of calories.

My "France 14" was likely the result of mostly the first two points I made about weight gain, but I might have spared myself at least a few of those pounds if I had been getting in my daily HIIT workout.

So why do I bring up minimal exercise here as a factor if it isn't a major one? Because it has myriad metabolic effects that offer wide-ranging benefits, from reduced stress to better brain health, which can kick-start a chain reaction of healthier habits. You may not see all of the changes immediately, but research shows that physical activity can increase neurogenesis (the creation of new nerve cells) and neuroplasticity, improve vascular function, lower inflammation, improve insulin sensitivity, and lessen your chances of suffering from stress-associated disorders, such as anxiety.

Let's Fix It: The #1 reason people use for not working out is lack of time. To help eliminate this excuse, Heather and I have brought in our longtime personal trainers to design DKFD-exclusive workouts. These workouts are the very same ones we follow, which means they are designed to be fast and efficient since we both lead very busy lives. No more excuses! Check out the workouts in Chapter 8.

Get Ready for Life with DKFD

I know I used my vacation weight gain as a springboard to talk about the problem of excess weight, but as a surgeon I feel an increased level of concern about this topic because there is absolutely no doubt that a patient's actual weight relative to their more "ideal" weight plays a key role in almost every aspect of the interaction between patient and surgeon. The list of potential problems is long:

* Determining proper doses of preoperative medications is more challenging on heavier patients as excess body fat can affect the accuracy of proper dosage calculations.
* Anesthesia itself is far riskier.
* Surgical dissection is more difficult and tedious and bloody.
* Healing can be compromised.
* Post-op recovery from early mobilization to ability to clear the lungs is more challenging.
* The results themselves are less consistent and effective.

And just in case you might see this list and think, "Well, I'm not ever going to get plastic surgery so this doesn't concern me," I bet you'd be hard-pressed to find a single surgeon in any specialty who disagrees with any of these points. I'm a specialist surgeon, so of course my focus is plastics, but these concerns are applicable to any situation in which you'd go under the knife.

Endurance is the key, not only to surgery but to everything in life; we are constantly being taxed and tested, and we never know when the hardest trials will arrive. Yet we can get ready for them. I often say that we can use today to make choices that will prepare us for whatever comes our way, even the unpredictable. You might not anticipate a situation in which you will be under the knife, but my philosophy is that you should give your body the best opportunity for success that you can. Making the choice to improve your

I've always shied away from high fat in my diet, thinking I'd gain weight. I'm loving this plan of eating high fat and protein. My blood sugar levels stay even during the day, I'm not HANGRY, no cravings, I'm satiated.

—ANGELA HILDRE RENNIE

health is about far more than just losing weight or looking good in a bikini; I see it as a dedication to greater life readiness.

It's never too late to learn how to take better care of yourself. The time is now to prime your metabolism for long-term success. In the Dubrow Keto Fusion Diet, we are going to show you how to do this in a way that is effective, enjoyable, and sustainable.

Heather's Hot Corner

The only thing that caught my eye here is the fact that Terry admitted to getting a little chunky while visiting the land of Champs-Élysées . . . I'm kidding! Truly, I think the most important takeaway from this chapter is that it's important to keep an open mind about change and opinions that may challenge the status quo, especially in the area of nutrition. I know personally I feel very much a product of the "diet-heart hypothesis" in that I still have a hard time breaking free of the "low-fat is best" mind-set, almost like I taught myself to think fat tastes bad. Yet I've discovered in exploring the land of full-fat foods a richness that I enjoy, and—guess what—they don't make me fat. Who knew?

I encourage you to be open to a similar change of heart—or mouth, really. In the pages ahead, you will discover how to do the DKFD, our plan to help you lose weight while gaining flavor. It's part keto, part low-carb, pure fusion. I know you're going to love it.

THE DKFD'S ULTIMATE FORMULA FOR SUSTAINABLE SUCCESS

The Dubrow Keto Fusion Diet: 12–8–4

The DKFD represents a blend of the best contemporary approaches to gaining metabolic control, an absolutely essential step if you want to achieve and maintain your ideal weight. We've fused together three strategies, which separately represent smart, powerful eating practices, and when joined together are made even better.

Like the Dubrow Diet, this program centers on the need to make adjustments in your eating schedule; *when* you eat really, truly matters a great deal when it comes to your metabolism.

The DKFD is based on a 12–8–4 daily eating schedule, meaning you'll stick to each of the strategies included for 12 hours, 8 hours, and 4 hours. Using this schedule as a structure, here's a quick look at how it all works (you'll get more on the science in the next two chapters, but this will help you get it at a glance!):

12 Reset

The DKFD starts off with a 12-hour Reset (aka fasting) window. This scheduled break from eating is based on the practice of intermittent fasting, which has proven to help people achieve reliable, targeted, and sustained weight loss, and activate autophagy, a self-cleaning internal process that can help combat cellular aging. It's successful because it prevents the production of insulin, which once released into the body can promote fat storage, prevent fat burning, and put the brakes on autophagy. No thank you, no thank you, no thank you.

In the DKFD, you may see us refer to intermittent fasting as *interval eating*; these are the same thing. You might wonder then why we call it interval eating? Well, it's simply because interval training is our favorite fitness method and we like the tidiness of thinking of how we eat and how we work out in terms of intervals.

You can incorporate the 12-hour Reset whenever it works best for you. This flexibility is one of the best things about eating according to schedule—it can easily be adjusted and customized if you work late hours or have any other type of atypical schedule. We tend to start our 12-hour Reset at 10 p.m. and carry it through to 10 a.m., and this is a schedule that will likely work for a lot of you who work traditional hours. However, you could easily have the Reset period from 8 p.m. to 8 a.m., 11 p.m. to 11 a.m.—whatever works for you!

When you get up in the morning, you will be able to have a few select items before your first official meal at the beginning of the 8-hour Recharge window. The select items during the 12-hour Reset period include water, coffee, tea, beet supplement drink, bouillon, bone broth, flavored sparkling water (without sugar), and greens-based supplement drink. You can also try out some of our Reset window–approved Consult Health Dubrow Keto/Fusion products such as the DKF Appetite Satiating Shake, and our crisps and bar.

See pages 78–81 for full list of what's allowed during the 12-hour Reset window.

8 Recharge

Once you've completed the 12-hour Reset, you'll enter the 8-hour Recharge window. This phase is a distinct addition to the DKFD—that is, it's not included in the Dubrow Diet—and is designed to extend the effects of fasting without extending the need to avoid eating. How cool is that?

This effect is made possible by eating a more ketogenic-based diet and keeping your carbohydrate intake selective and very low for 8 hours past your 12-hour Reset window. When you eat this way, you will continue to keep insulin production extremely low, thereby encouraging your body to burn fat for energy.

If you're scared of the ketogenic way of eating, you shouldn't be. We're both former keto doubters but realized that this wariness came largely from having no interest in being 24/7 hard-core keto eaters (which wouldn't be sustainable for us). As we mentioned in the introduction, what we've implemented here in the DKFD is a "liberalized keto," meaning you get more freedom to eat and enjoy your life more without having to swallow spoonfuls of oil.

What you will get to eat are some of our favorite meals like Salmon & Avocado Poke, Fat Bomb Burger Sliders, Cauliflower Bacon Hash, and Arugula Salad with Crispy Pan-Roasted Salmon. See?—more scrumptious than scary!

If we continue from the original timing of the 12-hour Reset window, this 8-hour Recharge window would then cover 10 a.m. to 6 p.m., the perfect hours during which to enjoy a hearty lunch and a snack, if you want, before moving into the final four.

See page 85 for full list of what's allowed during the 8-hour Recharge window.

4 Refuel

The last window of the DKFD is when the liberalized aspect of the diet really shows up. A traditional keto diet would require you to continue eating as you did in the 8-hour Recharge window, but we've included certain types of carbohydrates in this program so that you don't have to extend the more restrictive window beyond a more tenable timeframe.

The carbohydrates included are what are known as low-GI (glycemic index) carbs. The glycemic index is a system that assigns a number to a food based on how it impacts blood glucose levels. The more glucose in whatever you eat or drink, the more insulin your body produces in response. Remember, our goal is to keep insulin as low as possible to preserve a fat-burning environment rather than a fat-storing one.

Granted, the phrase "low-glycemic index" doesn't sound all that sexy, and even suggests foods that are maybe not too tasty, but the list of allowed low-GI carbs includes a lot of our favorite veggies: spinach, zucchini, broccoli, artichokes, butternut squash, bell peppers, and fennel, all of which can be cooked in flavorful oils made from olives, avocados (so good!), coconuts, walnuts, and more. You can enhance the oils with flavor boosters like herbs, spices, garlic,

I love that this diet allows a cheat day once a week. . . . It's motivating, and looking forward to that is what makes the diet sustainable. Plus the DKFD allows small amounts of healthy carbs during the week. This is what makes it a lifestyle!

—VERONICA GOMEZ

onion, and shallots. If you pair these with some of your favorite proteins, you will feel full and satisfied every time you eat. And there won't be the issue of flavorless food!

Now, again—you can incorporate this window whenever it works in your schedule; just make sure you get the 12-hour and 8-hour windows in back-to-back before digging into the foods allowed during the 4-hour Refuel timeframe. If you follow the sample schedule we've stuck to so far, your 4-hour Refuel window would occur from 6 p.m. to 10 p.m.

See page 94 for full list of what's allowed during the 4-hour Refuel window.

Putting 12–8–4 Together: A Week on the DKFD (If you like "free" stuff, you'll want to see this . . .)

So, that is your daily eating schedule on the Dubrow Keto Fusion Diet, and you will want to follow it for six consecutive days. On the seventh day, you will be treated to a free day—that's right, one with absolutely no eating schedule. No need to fast or keep an eye on the clock to figure out what you should be eating. After six days of DKFD eating, you deserve to take a break. Our only recommendation is to keep what you eat to 150 grams or fewer carbs; otherwise your cells will have to fight harder to get back into fat-burning mode.

CHAPTER 3

THE FABULOUS EFFECT OF FASTING COMBINED WITH EATING FATS

We've identified that an overreliance on carbs is one of the main factors behind the metabolic dysfunction plaguing most people today. We also believe that this dysfunction could be a primary cause of insulin resistance, type 2 diabetes, obesity, and the related systemic inflammation that can set you up to develop heart disease and other serious health issues.

If you're wondering if this is a conclusion that's unique to the Dubrow Keto Fusion Diet, it's not. Research published in the journal *Cell Metabolism* in May 2017 showed that "insulin resistance has evolved to become generally accepted as the predominant factor leading to type 2 diabetes, and the most probable single link among a constellation of cardiometabolic risk factors known as the metabolic syndrome linking obesity, type 2 diabetes and cardiovascular disease."

If the problem is that most people are eating too many factory carbs, then the solution should be to just stop eating these foods, right? Well, that's a significant part of the solution, but it's not all there is to it. Before we get to that and the science of smarter carb selection, you have to first perform what I think of as a metabolic reconstruction.

Don't worry—you will not be required to go under the knife for this procedure, nor will what you have to do be painful. Reconstructing your metabolism is purely about making selective, simple, and effective dietary changes that will do all the internal work for you.

In this chapter, we are going to look at two of these changes incorporated in the 12-hour Reset and 8-hour Recharge windows: fasting and eating a fat-rich diet, respectively. Even though the fusion (of Dubrow Keto *Fusion* Diet fame) has three parts, these first two should be seen as having the tightest bond; in fact, we want you to consider them an inseparable pair—wherever your Reset window goes, your Recharge window will always follow. When you keep these two locked together, you ensure that you will get the absolute most metabolic benefits possible from the DKFD.

The Return of the Metabolic Miracle Worker

In *The Dubrow Diet*, we referred to fasting as a "metabolic miracle worker," and this only slightly exaggerated moniker remains just as appropriate now as it was then. That is to say, there hasn't been any sort of scientific switcheroo about the powerful effects fasting can have on cellular function. In fact, research only continues to prove the benefits of "willing abstinence or reduction from some or all food, drink, or both, for a period of time." (I'm a fan of this definition because it offers an important reminder—this is a *willing* practice implemented with a specific purpose!)

As you know, you will practice a 12-hour fast during the Reset window, and during this time you will eat or drink only from a short list of approved items (see list on page 78). Let's look at what fasting is, why we love it so much, and why it's been carried over into the DKFD.

The Basics of Fasting

Fasting has long been considered a reliable method for initiating a reset or reboot of systems, both physical and spiritual in nature. In fact, many popular religions incorporate some type of fasting—in Judaism, people fast on Yom Kippur; Muslims fast daily for an entire month during Ramadan; and Christians practice selective fasting by eliminating something during the forty days of Lent. In each case, the fast is intended to create a certain level of clarity and enhanced spiritual connection.

Fasting for physiological reasons is believed to be nearly as old as if not older than fasting in religious traditions. As far back as the first century, the famous Greek philosopher Plutarch wrote, "Instead of using medicine, better fast today." Much later on in the sixteenth century, the Swiss physician Paracelsus suggested that the idea of a voluntary and temporary abstinence from caloric intake was a way to activate the "physical within."

Now, I'm not one to just go around praising medical opinions from the past, whether they're from decades or centuries ago, but these guys were ahead of their time and right on the money with their proclamations. Contemporary research has linked the practice of fasting with reduced risk of developing type 2 diabetes, heart disease, and certain neurological disorders, and it's also been shown to potentially delay the development of cancerous tumors. Oh, and it's been proven to be a bona fide fat killer, which means maybe it should also be considered the plastic surgeon within? I definitely like the sound of that.

It's hard to believe that taking a break from eating can do so much, but in the words of *this* doctor, it's the real deal. To understand why it's so effective, you have to understand a little about the basics of metabolism, and especially the role of the primary players, glucose and insulin.

The simplest way to look at metabolism is to see it as a process of conversion—the foods you eat and the beverages you drink are converted by your cells into fuel that can be used within the body to power all your internal systems. How exactly each food or beverage is converted depends upon its macronutrient classification, which is to say it depends upon whether you've eaten a carbohydrate, a protein, a fat, or something that's a mixture of all three. Each of these macronutrients is processed differently by the body.

Carbohydrates are broken down into glucose. This includes all types of carbohydrates—processed carbs such as chips and cookies; complex carbs such as brown rice and sweet potatoes; fibrous carbs such as broccoli and asparagus. If it's available, your cells will preferentially choose glucose over any other source of fuel. Why? Because it burns fast, like kindling in a fire, and your body is smart; it's not going to work harder than it has to to keep itself up and running.

Once glucose is in your bloodstream, it's referred to as blood glucose or blood sugar, and it is ready for use. However, it can't be put to work all on its own; glucose needs insulin to help it get into your cells. And this is why in typical carbohydrate metabolism, the presence of blood sugar will stimulate insulin production in the pancreas and the insulin will go right to work unlocking your cells and ushering glucose in. Once inside the cells, any glucose that's needed immediately gets used. If this were the end of the story, everything would be fine; it's what happens next that can program your body to store and save fat.

The biological reality is that your body only has so much immediate need for glucose. After your cells have utilized what they need, they'll bond any remaining glucose molecules together to form glycogen (which is basically like a group hug of glucose molecules), to be stored in the liver for future use. And once your liver is at glycogen capacity, any remaining glucose molecules get converted to fat.

You may wonder why this excess glucose isn't just flagged as waste and excreted out of the body. Because your body is interested in one thing and one thing only, and that is survival. Your cells wouldn't dare waste such a valuable life-sustaining resource as glucose, because as far as they know, there is no guaranteed meal on the horizon. In fact, your body is so committed to saving these reserves that it won't even touch the glucose that's been stored as fat if you introduce new glucose, that is, carbs, into your diet on the daily. Why would it trek all the way to your liver for energy that it has to convert back into glucose, by the way, when you've just handed it some fast-and-easy fuel?

If you consistently eat a high-carb diet, you essentially get stuck on this fat-storage cycle. It's made even worse if the carbohydrates you're eating are the processed, factory variety— these cause rapid spikes in blood sugar that call for equally rapid rises in insulin. Repeated rapid rises in insulin can in turn contribute to a number of problems, including:

❋ **The inability to burn fat.** When insulin is present, stored fat from your tissues will not be used as energy. Plain and simple.

❋ **Insulin resistance.** If your diet creates a high-blood sugar + high-insulin environment, your cells can grow tired of insulin knocking at the door constantly, saying, "Glucose fuel delivery," and eventually start to ignore it. When this happens, your blood sugar remains high along with the concentration of insulin, both of which contribute to systemic inflammation and in most cases lead eventually to type 2 diabetes if left unaddressed.

Proteins, on the other hand, are metabolized differently. In the same way that carbs are made up of glucose, proteins are made up of amino acids. When you eat protein-rich foods (such as fish, chicken, whey, etc.), they get broken down by enzymes in the stomach and converted to amino acids, which are then absorbed into the small intestines and sent back out into the body to do the job of repairing muscles and building tissue and providing the raw materials from which hormones can be made.

I know this may make protein sound like the ideal food, and it is in many ways a quality macronutrient. There is one reason, however, that you have to keep your protein intake right around moderate instead of high—and this reason is gluconeogenesis. I know you're probably thinking, "Ah, the old gluconeogenesis issue . . ."

Well, maybe you're not thinking it now, but you're going to be soon.

When I talked about carbohydrate metabolism, I mentioned the matter of excess glucose getting stored as fat. The thing about protein is that when you eat too much of it— again more than your cells can use—it will get converted into glucose and then, *bam*, insulin is released, and you're back to storing any surplus glucose as fat. Research has shown that a "normal" protein intake will prevent amino acids being converted to glucose, which is why on the DKFD you don't want to overdo it on protein.

Fats are a whole different ball of metabolic wax that I'll get into in greater detail on page 47. For now, it's enough to understand that fats in foods are broken down in the body to fatty acids, which get metabolized through a long series of chemical reactions and ultimately end up getting used to help repair cells, fight infection, lubricate joints and nerves, and more. Fats take the longest for your body to metabolize, which is why they will keep you fuller longer compared to carbs and protein.

Most important, fats do not get converted to glucose, which means they can only ever moderately stimulate the production of insulin.

The Advantages of an Insulin-Free Morning

When you wake up in the morning, your cortisol levels are naturally increased to help get you going. As soon as you introduce any glucose source and insulin appears, cortisol and insulin begin to work together to help increase your fat stores. So when you keep insulin out of the picture in the mornings, you prevent the "fat-accumulating couple" of insulin and cortisol from spending time together.

OK, finally, now that you've been so patient in sitting through Dr. Dubrow's Metabolism 101 class, I can tell you how the Reset period and its focus on fasting works in relation to all this.

As I said at the beginning, fasting is all about the primary players involved in metabolism: glucose and insulin. Or rather, it's all about making these *no longer* the primary players. We've established that the combined effect of glucose and insulin in excess contributes to weight gain and a whole host of other problems.

Here's a play-by-play of what happens when you fast:

* With the help of insulin, your cells utilize any glucose that's remaining and readily available.
* Your cells then dig deeper for glucose, and burn through any that's stored in the liver as glycogen.
* Your cells dig deeper still and seek out any excess protein that can be converted to glucose via gluconeogenesis.
* Finally, once glucose is exhausted, and as your body's need for fuel continues, it will begin to seek out alternative sources. (Lucky for us, the next preferred source in line is fat, aka fatty acids, aka the excess fatty tissue you'd probably like to eliminate—and the sole purpose of you reading this book!) A biochemist might describe this fat-seeking process as mobilizing and oxidizing fatty acids, but I like to just say that at this stage your body has literally started to burn stored fat for energy. You have reached what's known as ketosis, which is when your cells have shifted to using ketones for fuel instead of glucose.
* As ketone levels rise in the body, they replace glucose as the primary energy source.

A Metabolic Mouthful

Glucose, gluconeogenesis, insulin, ketones . . . there are a lot of words floating around here that might have made your eyes glaze over and your brain go numb (at least, that's usually Heather's response when I start to wander too far down the metabolism science rabbit hole). If you're like her and you want the ten-second summary, here it is:

When you have an overreliance on carbs, your blood sugar (glucose) regularly rises, requiring insulin production. Insulin allows for cellular energy to be used, but it can also lead to increased fat storage. If you want a fat-burning environment instead, you must eliminate the presence of insulin, which first requires an absence of glucose. To create low- to no-glucose levels, you essentially have to remove all carbs from your diet forever; or if you want to be a bit more civilized about it, you can rely on a combined strategy that first burns through any glucose that's in the body, then, second, shifts you to burn stored fat (ketones, baby!), and, third, keeps glucose low enough that any that's generated is used immediately instead of stored.

This is what the DKFD is designed to help you do.

Of course, you probably already know the words *ketosis* and *ketones* because they're related to the ketogenic diet. *Ketogenic* simply means "ketone producing." Following a ketogenic diet will help you produce ketones, which in turn marks a shift toward burning fat. And this is why you'll be part-time keto on this plan, but the fastest way to get to a ketotic state is by fasting. In "The Effect of Short-Term Fasting on Liver and Skeletal Muscle Lipid, Glucose, and Energy Metabolism in Healthy Women and Men," a study that was published in the *Journal of Lipid Research*, researchers determined that ketogenic diets can increase ketones fourfold, while fasting can increase ketones by up to twentyfold.

This is why the Reset window comes first—it's the fast track to fat burning. There is a long list of additional advantages to shifting your cells and body to run even part-time off ketones, and I'll address these in the next section, starting on page 47. But before I get to that, I want to first acknowledge the other beneficial side effects of fasting:

Lowered inflammation: Research has revealed that when you take an extended break from eating, a compound called ß-hydroxybutyrate is produced. This compound has been shown to block the beginning of an inflammatory response that's often involved in atherosclerosis and diseases such as type 2 diabetes and Alzheimer's.

Fasting also reduces oxidative stress, the everyday wear and tear caused by keeping the engine of your body running 24/7, which can damage cells and lead to chronic inflammation. Oxidative stress and chronic inflammation play major roles in the development of almost all age-related diseases. This effect alone should put fasting first on your list as an approach to health. *But there's more.*

Reduced risk for heart disease and stroke: Pressing pause on eating can lower blood pressure, reduce insulin resistance, and increase insulin sensitivity, all of which are big-time wins for heart health. When your cells develop resistance to insulin (typically due to an overreliance on carbs), big problems, including a disturbance of fat metabolism, start brewing. The type of disturbance I'm talking about is one that can result in high triglycerides, low levels of high-density lipoprotein (aka HDL, the good cholesterol), and the introduction of small, dense low-density lipoproteins (aka LPA, the very bad cholesterol). This trio is a killer and consistently linked with coronary artery disease.

Improved glucose control: Developing research has found that intermittent fasting can help improve glucose response, even in people who are at risk of type 2 diabetes. This means that when you do eat carbs, your body will only get better at metabolizing them.

Chromium Power

We are borderline obsessed with researching ways to create better carbo-hydrate metabolism. And in most cases, we've found that the best "tools" for improvement are diet-based. But there is one supplement, the essential trace element chromium, that seems to have the ability to get into the mo-lecular mix of things when carbohydrates, glucose, and insulin are involved.

Some studies in animals have shown that chromium can improve insulin sensitivity. Other research has found that it has several positive effects on the metabolic pathways involving carbohydrate metabolism. This includes helping your cells better absorb glucose, which can mean a need for less insulin, and improving overall insulin responsiveness. Chromium can also help regulate oxidative stress and inflammation by inhibiting the produc-tion of certain pro-inflammatory proteins. For these reasons (and because it doesn't have adverse effects), it continues to be explored for its potential role in helping improve metabolism for people with type 2 diabetes.

You can try including chromium in your daily supplements; a good starter dose is about 500 micrograms per day. You can also check out our Du-brow Keto/Fusion Carb-ology supplement, which includes 500 micrograms of chromium along with some other specialized plant ingredients that help minimize rapid elevations of insulin after carbohydrate consumption (I like to call these capsules my little "carb crushers").

Of course, never start taking supplements without your physician's ap-proval!

Boosted all-around anti-aging and anti-disease effects: One of the coolest and most rewarding benefits of taking a voluntary break from eating is increased autophagy. If you've ever lis-tened to our podcast or if you read our book *The Dubrow Diet,* you know I'm pretty much autophagy's #1 fan. Autophagy is essentially a cellular cleanup process during which your cells break down and recycle or get rid of any sort of toxic metabolic clutter left lying around within your internal environment. When this clutter is left in place for too long, it can interfere in metabolic interactions and lead to the type of molecular dysfunction that serves as the foundation of disease. Think of it this way: If you don't vacuum your house, the dust starts to build up on the floors. You then start to breathe in dust, and bringing in toxins is bound to affect your long-term health. Autophagy is the vacuuming of your cells.

This process has gotten a ton of well-earned attention in the areas of anti-aging and disease prevention. It actually received worldwide recognition in 2016 when Japanese cell biologist Yoshinori Ohsumi won the Nobel Prize for his molecular discoveries related to this intelligent self-cleaning process. Since then, autophagy has been noted for its role in decreasing chronic inflammation and specifically inflammation in the brain, where autophagy's anti-inflammatory effect could help protect against neurodegenerative disorders such as Alzheimer's.

The future of autophagy is incredibly promising. I think someday soon we'll see that molecular scientists have designed a pill or patch or implant that will increase autophagy and hopefully prevent or slow down the effects of cognitive diseases and cancer. The good news is you don't have to wait for any pill to hit the market; you can practice fasting and amp up autophagy all on your own. Since the process of autophagy naturally declines as we age, the sooner you start activating it, the better the long-term effects will be.

These are some of the potential benefits when you commit to a Reset each day. If you want to *extend* these benefits even further (and add on a few more), you will follow this Reset period with a strategic Recharge period. In the DKFD, Recharge is an 8-hour period of time that you dedicate to eating a higher-fat diet. When you eat a fat-rich diet immediately after fasting, you continue to take advantage of the fat-burning, health-promoting internal environment you've just created.

Let's explore further why this pairing is powerful.

First Comes Fasting, Then Comes Fat

You know now that the approach to eating on this plan is built around the goal of increasing your body's natural ability to burn fat. We accomplish this by programming your cells to use any available glucose for energy, whether it's in the food you've eaten or sourced from glycogen stored in your liver; dropping the fat-storage hormone insulin to near undetectable levels; and shifting fuel use to stored fat, that is, ketones.

Ideally, you want to stay in this space where your system is running off ketones for energy for as long as possible. The primary difficulty many people experience when they go "full-keto" is that they're grossed out by eating so much fat for such an extended period. As evidenced by watching Natalie swig oils, well, we know it's just not sustainable—which is why in the DKFD, you'll eat a higher-fat diet combined with a small amount of low-GI carbs (more on why this type only in the next chapter) for just 8 hours. This is what we've found to be the just-right duration; you get a significant percentage of the benefits of keto without the unpleasant, unpalatable parts.

There's a lot of research that's shown that ketones can produce both unnoticeable (internal) and noticeable (more external or experimental) benefits. Here are some of the standouts:

* Ketones will help protect your brain by turning up production of a protein called brain-derived neurotrophic factor (BDNF). BDNF can help make your mitochondria more resistant to cellular stress and enhance neuroprotection.

* Ketones can help turn up chemical anti-inflammatory pathways within the body while simultaneously turning down those that cause inflammation. Molecular science researchers have described how this happens as an "intricate molecular waltz." In the simplest terms, ketones seem to have a way to suppress inflammatory genes.

* Ketones may help improve cholesterol levels. Some studies in obese people have shown that a ketogenic type of diet can lower triglycerides and LDL cholesterol, and increase the level of HDL cholesterol.

And on the noticeable front . . .

* Ketones have been referred to as a super fuel because they produce more adenosine triphosphate (ATP, which is the molecular currency of our cells) compared to glucose. For you, this can translate to feeling better brainwise—that is, you might notice that you can think more clearly or that you feel just generally sharper.

* Ketones keep you fuller longer than glucose. A study titled "Ketosis, Ketogenic Diet and Food Intake Control: A Complex Relationship" found that ketones appear capable of influencing biochemical signals that help control your appetite (researchers writing in this study described ketones as contributing to a "hunger-reduction phenomenon").

* Of course, I'm sure you're also interested in knowing that running off ketones instead of glucose has proven to be *very* effective in promoting weight loss.

When you shift your body to use ketones as fuel, you are taking advantage of your innate internal system built to help you survive. Our ancestors' bodies needed to run off glucose or ketones; if they hadn't, they couldn't have survived times of limited food or famine for days. While we've come a long way from the hunter-gatherer days, our metabolic systems really haven't changed all that much; we're just cavemen and cavewomen in nicer clothing.

The good news is that we don't have to go back to those much tougher times to tap into this metabolic adaptation. Nor do we have to create survivalist scenarios—we can manipulate our metabolism to burn fat for us.

An important part of staying in this fat-burning mode is eating fat, and probably a bit more than you're used to. It sounds counterintuitive to eat fat to burn fat, but remember: You want to keep insulin out of the picture and prevent the fat-storage cycle from getting up and running. Eating fat also provides your body with fatty acids, which are converted in the liver to ketones to be used as energy. Dietary fats also help your body absorb fat-soluble vitamins A, D, and E, and they provide the raw materials from which hormones such as estrogen and testosterone are made.

While following the DKFD, you'll prioritize healthy fats whenever you're eating (and not fasting). There are two rules to keep in mind as you work to incorporate more fats into your diet:

1. **This isn't a fat-eating free-for-all:** Eating too much of anything can lead to weight gain. This is why you will eat strategically to avoid the problem of overnutrition, that is, consistently consuming more calories than your body needs. It's surprisingly easy to cut your calorie intake when you focus on fat—it's so much more filling than carbs and even pro-

tein that you will experience a natural, healthy decline in appetite, and in turn likely eat fewer calories without even noticing.

2. **Not all fats are created equal:** You will want to focus on eating high-quality fats as much as possible. A lot of dietary fats contain a mix of types of fat but will be categorized by the type of fat of which they have the most. On the DKFD, you'll want to focus on eating saturated fats and unsaturated fats, both monounsaturated and polyunsaturated, and avoiding trans fats. What follows is a little more about the different fats.

Saturated Fats

Saturated fats are found mostly in animal products such as beef, chicken, turkey, lamb, eggs, bacon, and butter, and nutrient-rich oils such as coconut oil and medium-chain triglyceride (MCT) oil. Most are solid at room temperature (and quite tasty). They are called saturated because they are formed by carbon bonds that are attached to or "saturated" by hydrogen atoms.

Saturated fats have been a source of confusion for several decades. Are they good, bad, somewhere in between? A consensus has been a moving target.

In Chapter 1, I mentioned how saturated fats were painted as the villain in heart health as far back as the 1950s. This was thanks to the diet-heart hypothesis, which suggested that saturated fats increased cholesterol and then caused heart disease. Beginning in 1977, this theory went on to shape the dietary habits of the nation despite a lack of definitive proof. Almost forty years later, an evaluation of several studies (called a metastudy or meta-analysis, and in this case specifically titled "Evidence from Randomised Controlled

Trials Did Not Support the Introduction of Dietary Fat Guidelines in 1977 and 1983: A Systematic Review and Meta-Analysis") on the relationship between saturated fat, cholesterol, and heart disease acknowledged the premature nature of the government-issued advice: "Government dietary fat recommendations were untested in any trial prior to being introduced."

I often talk about the changing tides of research, especially when it comes to an isolated element such as caffeine or, in this case, fat. But I think the more recent scientific studies will speak to a positive directional trend on the topic of saturated fats:

* One 2015 study published in the *American Journal of Clinical Nutrition* determined that saturated fats are not associated with cardiovascular disease, stroke, or type 2 diabetes.
* Another piece, published in November 2017 and called "Associations of Fats and Carbohydrate Intake with Cardiovascular Disease and Mortality in 18 Countries from Five Continents (PURE): A Prospective Cohort Study," found that a high carb intake and not high fat intake was "associated with higher risk of total mortality." Total fat and individual types of fat were conversely "related to lower total mortality."
* High carbohydrate intake also seems to increase an unfavorable cholesterol profile across the board, including raising levels of small, dense particles of cholesterol. These particles, known clinically as low-density lipoproteins, are the little destructive devils you want to watch out for; they're like hard, chemically destabilized, sticky "BBs" that can penetrate arterial walls, creating indentations where dangerous plaque can develop. And this is why they've been noted as a better marker for prediction of cardiovascular disease than other types of cholesterol.

Based on developments such as these, I encourage you to surrender any lingering fears of saturated fat and enjoy eating healthy varieties (you'll find the best sources in the Food Lists in Chapter 5). Of course, since I am not your doctor, you should discuss any dietary change you want to make with your personal physician. And if you're curious or concerned, you might consider having a cholesterol panel run four to six weeks after starting the diet to see how your body is responding to an increase in fat intake.

The ABCs of MCT

If you've heard anything about keto, you've likely heard talk of something called MCT (short for medium-chain triglyceride, aka medium-chain fatty acid) oil. What is it? And why do keto fanatics love it so much? Well, I'm glad you asked . . . because the answer will offer a little more understanding on how fat metabolism works.

Warning: Chemistry crash course ahead!

All fats are made up of fatty acids, which are chains of carbon molecules (a "triglyceride" happens when two carbon bonds link up with a compound called a glycerol and they become a party of three). The description of a fat depends upon the length of the carbon chain:

* **Short-chain fatty acids** contain fewer than 6 carbon atoms and are produced in the body. Fibrous foods such as artichokes, asparagus, garlic, and apples can increase production of these acids.

* **Medium-chain fatty acids** have between 6 and 12 carbon atoms and are distinct because of how they are metabolized. MCTs are broken down directly in the liver and converted to ketones for immediate use, which is why they're less likely to get stored as fat. In studies, MCTs have been shown to help promote weight loss. You'll find the most MCTs in coconut oil and some in palm oil and dairy foods such as butter, cheese,

milk, and yogurt. Of course, the purest form you can get is MCT oil, which is 100 percent MCT.

* **Long-chain fatty acids** have between 13 and 21 carbon atoms and make up the most commonly consumed fat type in the Western diet (likely because they're found in the types of oils often used in processed foods). Some of the highest concentrations of long-chain fatty acids are found in safflower and sunflower oils, and in pork, beef, organ meats, and egg yolks. They're also in coconut and palm oils, other nut and seed oils, and fish and fish oil.

It's easy to see the ketogenic appeal in MCT oil. The downside, however, is that swallowing a spoonful of pure oil is not my cup of tea—although I don't mind a little of it *in* tea or coffee (see our coffee recipes starting on page 110).

Unsaturated Fats

Unsaturated fats are liquid at room temperature, and they are called "un"-saturated because they contain fewer hydrogen atoms than saturated fats. The two types of unsaturated fat, monounsaturated and polyunsaturated, are separated by the number of bonds they contain (mono = one; poly = multiple). These types of fats are found mostly in plant-based sources, although they exist in fish as well. Mono- and polyunsaturated fats vary in stability, which means that they can tolerate different levels of heat and exposure before becoming oxidized or rancid.

Monounsaturated fats (MUFAs) are found in olives; avocados; nuts such as almonds, hazelnuts, and macadamias; seeds such as sesame and pumpkin; and the oils made from any of these foods. These are considered relatively stable fats so you can cook with them at low to medium heats and they won't get too disrupted, chemically speaking.

Monounsaturated fats have been shown in animal studies to increase calcium concentrations in bone, and in people they have proven effective at creating better absorption of vitamin D.

Polyunsaturated fats (PUFAs) are found mostly in plant-sourced oils such as corn, cottonseed, flax, safflower, sesame, soybean, and walnut oil. PUFAs also occur naturally in fish. Polyunsaturated fats are divided into two types, omega-3 and omega-6, and most of them contain some of each type. Your body needs both types to function at its best, but far less omega-6. The problem is omega-6 oils are the ones that are more prevalent, especially in processed foods; just about any type of packaged cookie, chip, cracker, etc., will contain soybean, safflower, or corn oil. These might sound harmless, but omega-6 fats can trigger signaling molecules that increase inflammation.

Omega-3 fats, on the other hand, are anti-inflammatory and can help lower total cholesterol. The goal then when con-

I love that I'm in control—when I eat, what I eat, how much I eat. I like that I'm changing my body to where it's no longer struggling during the "fast" but actually looking forward to it, and I feel myself recharging during that time. It's not easy, but it's definitely a balance of effort and reward—more so than any other, more restrictive diet plan.

—ANIA BEDNARCZYK

suming PUFAs is to be selective and opt for those that provide more omega-3s than omega-6s. Walnuts, flax, and fish and other seafood are some of the best choices.

Trans Fats

It's widely known at this point that trans fats are bad, but we can't get into the topic of dietary fat without mentioning these bad guys. Seriously, if this were a movie, trans fats would be the villain. Artificial trans fats are created when vegetable oils are hydrogenated, and they are the most processed type of fat you can find. Even though they've been banned by the FDA, you might still find them lurking in foods such as microwave popcorn, margarine, vegetable shortening, fast foods, and boxed baked goods.

Trans fats have been linked to increased risk of heart disease, type 2 diabetes, and systemic inflammation. Importantly, research has also shown that these types of fats are "unable to stimulate an autophagic response." Remember, you want autophagy to occur so you can benefit from its anti-aging, disease-fighting effects!

In the Food Lists in Chapter 5, you'll get more detail on what specific fat-rich foods you'll want to focus on in the DKFD. Overall, you will get the most benefit from any dietary fats when you get them from quality, fresh foods that will feed your body with the most nutrients and natural antioxidants and fuel your metabolic ketone production. Stay away from processed and fried foods, which are often full of destabilized fatty acids ready to damage your cells as soon as they enter your body.

Heather's Hot Corner

As a mom of twins, I love dynamic duos and power couples, which is why I've become such a huge fan of fasting combined with eating dietary fats. Pairing the two seems to have a pretty cool metabolic effect, and may help initiate the kind of fat burning you want to happen if weight loss is your goal.

When you first begin pairing up these two, don't overthink it—you're going to fast for 12 hours and then when you eat during the next 8 hours, you'll want to focus on nutrient-rich fats and a limited carb intake. What specific foods should you eat? You'll find out in the Food Lists in Chapter 5.

CHAPTER 4

CHOOSING BETTER CARBS, OR WHY LOW-CARB IS SO LAST YEAR

When physicians began using a dietary approach to help treat seizures in epileptic patients, they used a strict ketogenic diet. Transitioning the body to run off ketones proved to be an effective and powerful tool against the neuronal instability that initiates seizures in the brain. But strict keto meant eating a diet that consisted of *90 percent fat*. Even in sick, very motivated people, this often proved too tough to follow. Over time, different forms of the ketogenic diet with varying macronutrient percentages were developed with the goal of producing a diet that was more sustainable.

One of those variations was something called the low-glycemic index treatment (LGIT) diet. This approach was developed in 2002 and is based on the idea that the introduction of *some* carbs would make the diet easier to follow and more enjoyable.

Now, it couldn't be just any carbs—it had to be low-glycemic carbs, which have less of an effect on blood sugar and therefore prevent the type of dramatic fluctuations in glucose that activate high insulin production. In a small initial study, this "liberalized keto" diet proved successful in helping people reduce seizures by up to 90 percent (you can read more about this in the study, which was published in the journal *Neurology* under the title "Low-Glycemic-

Index Treatment: A Liberalized Ketogenic Diet for Treatment of Intractable Epilepsy").

I explored the metabolic science of this approach further and determined it was the missing link in the fusion. Since our goal was to eliminate the presence of excess glucose + excess insulin, while still creating a diet that people could stay on, adding the right kind of carbs was the key. Low-glycemic carbs could significantly minimize the fat-storage cycle associated with factory carbs, and also help resolve associated problems such as increased inflammation, risk for type 2 diabetes and other diseases, and weight gain. When fused with fasting plus a period of keto eating, it would prove to be an ideal, even enjoyable fat-killer combo.

In this chapter, I'll give you a quick rundown on low-GI carbs, how they're metabolized in the body, and when you'll want to eat them.

The "Slow-Release Carb" Enters the Picture

The glycemic index initially came about in 1981 when Canadian doctor and nutrition scientist David Jenkins and his colleagues were trying to understand the impact of carbohydrates on diabetes. At the time, it was known that all carbohydrates had 4 calories per gram, but what was not understood was why the body seemed to respond to the same amount of various carbs differently. Their research revealed that the response differed based on the glycemic response, or the amount of blood sugar that had entered the bloodstream after a food was eaten.

With this information, they designed the glycemic index, which assigned a food a specific number ranging from 1 to 100 based on the rise in blood sugar it produced. Less glucose equaled lower numbers; more glucose equaled higher numbers. There were low-, medium-, and high-GI foods; the lower the GI, the healthier it is.

There are a lot of factors that influence where a food falls on the glycemic index: What type of starch it contains, how much fiber it has, and whether the food also has some fat and/or protein can all impact the GI number it's assigned. Each of these can directly determine how fast or slowly your blood sugar rises (and how extreme of a spike in insulin is required). Low-GI carbohydrates, many of which are nonstarchy and contain fiber, have also been called "slow-release carbs," which I love—it's an easy way to almost visualize a food's effect in your body.

Here's a snapshot of each glycemic index category:

LOW-GI FOODS

* Assigned a GI number between 1 and 55
* Higher in fiber and low in starch
* Promote a slower rise in blood sugar
* Examples: most fruits; intact grains such as barley, bulgur, and brown rice; nonstarchy vegetables

MEDIUM-GI FOODS

* Assigned a GI number between 56 and 69
* Low in fiber and high in starch
* Promote a faster rise in blood sugar
* Examples: white rice, corn, pasta, cereals containing refined wheat, potatoes (including sweet potatoes)

HIGH-GI FOODS

* Assigned a GI number of 70 or higher
* Pretty much no fiber and all starch
* Promote a very rapid rise in blood sugar

* Examples: bagels, cakes, donuts, white bread, rice cakes, most packaged cereals

I want to tell you to avoid everything in the medium- and high-GI categories, but who are we kidding—life would be a bit of a bummer without corn, potatoes, or white rice every once in a while. You can dip your toe into the medium zone occasionally—just make sure it's on a cheat day. But you really should eliminate high-GI foods on the DKFD as they will interfere with your progress (one good cheat for this is our "Invisible Rice," page 177, which is prepared in a way to reduce the glycemic response). A long-term elimination is also recommended as these foods are linked to several health issues that can have very serious consequences affecting quality and duration of life, including increased risk for heart disease and weight gain, and are considered to have a "robust association" with type 2 diabetes. Developing research has shown that foods promoting a high glycemic response may also contribute to female infertility, colorectal cancer, and age-related macular degeneration.

On the flip side, low-GI foods are the highest quality carbohydrates you can consume, and they have so much to offer your health and metabolism.

The Benefits of Staying Low

Before we get into why low-GI foods are so awesome, I just want to address some of you out there who may be yawning or rolling your eyes at the undeniable lack of pizzazz in all this glycemic index talk—we get it; it's not sexy or tabloid worthy. But I'm telling you, even though it sounds dull, it will without a doubt help transform your internal environment and ensure phenomenal results on this program. With that being said, let's jump back to the positive effects of low-glycemic index foods. These include:

A stable metabolism and limited carb cravings. When you stick to eating in a way that produces only a low and slow increase in glucose levels, you essentially give your cells time to greet increased blood sugar in a measured way. Insulin will be triggered, but not in excess—more a trickle than a downpour. This entire, more civilized brand of metabolism will set you up to have a stable appetite (i.e., free of intense cravings for factory carbs) and even energy levels.

A quicker return to using ketones for fuel. For our purposes on the DKFD, keeping glucose low is extremely important, since when glucose is present, ketones (stored fat) will not be used for energy. If you limit your carb intake to low-GI carbs, this should help drive your metabolism into ketosis more quickly during your Reset and Recharge windows.

Fewer negative side effects typically associated with keto-type diets. Plenty of people have tried pure ketogenic diets and experienced some positive results, but they've had to feel miserable along the way. However, we've found that when you combine a keto-ish diet with low-GI, slow-digesting carbs that have less impact on insulin, you get the good without the bad.

The diet has eliminated cravings; after dinner I no longer crave late-night snacks. The interval fasting/eating is so much easier than it sounds.

—MICHELLE RAMON

Since one of the primary goals of the DKFD is to get your metabolism into a fat-burning state, we've incorporated a little extra strategy into our brand of low-GI eating. This is introduced as a way to help ensure your fat-burning window lasts as long as possible.

What we've done is stripped down the 8-hour Recharge window to include only the lowest of the low-GI foods and suggested that you keep your intake to 15 grams or fewer of these carbs during this 8-hour window. And we've saved any foods that will promote a more significant rise in glucose for the 4-hour Refuel window. This means saving fruits and approved grains and certain starchier vegetables for the evenings.

In addition to low-GI carbs, we've also highlighted during Refuel an additional type of carbohydrate, something called a resistant starch. Resistant starches digest in a different way from other types of carbohydrates, and because of this have been classified as "unavailable carbohydrates" (Heather likes to call these invisible carbs!). Instead of being processed in the large intestine and raising glucose, they're digested in the small intestines where they essentially ferment like a fine wine and increase the population of good bacteria. This makes them incredibly good for your digestion. Resistant starches can help lower cholesterol, alleviate constipation, and increase fullness, making meals more satisfying.

While you might have heard suggestions to avoid carbs at night, research suggests that this is precisely when you *should* be eating them. In the study "Greater Weight Loss and Hormonal Changes After 6 Months Diet with Carbohydrates Eaten Mostly at Dinner," researchers compared two groups of dieters who were told to eat the same number of calories, but the only difference was that one group could eat carbs all day and the other had to limit their carb intake to the evenings. What they found was that eating carbohydrates with dinner helped improve glucose response, and cholesterol markers, and resulted in an overall increased sense of appetite satisfaction during the day. This group also lost more weight, more overall fat, and more abdominal fat than those who ate carbs throughout the day.

The other cool thing that happens when you eat specifically low-GI carbs at night is that you can improve your cells' response to glucose the following day; this strategic type of eating seems to have positive carryover effects that create a pattern of metabolic success.

When you get to the Food Lists in Chapter 5, you'll see dozens of filling and flavorful carbs fit for consumption on the DKFD. Some you'll want to save for the 4-hour Refuel window given their carbohydrate grams. Overall, I think you'll be pleasantly surprised to see the variety and number of options. Be sure to check out the recipes Heather and I have created exclusively for this book that feature some delicious ways to enjoy low-GI carbs (don't miss one of my favorites: Southern-Style Shrimp & Cauliflower "Grits," page 137).

Heather's Hot Corner

There's no question that some carbs are better for you than others; you *know* this without Terry or me telling you. You know that chips and cookies and candy are probably not the best thing for you if you want to achieve good health. But that doesn't mean it's easy to stop eating these tasty little devils. So how do you do it? Well, you first consider the consequences of keeping them in your diet, which include challenges with weight, greater risk for disease, and generally feeling a little bit like crap most of the time. Then you become a bit of a carb snob—sorry, only low-GI carbs for me, darling. Demand better for yourself because it's better for your health!

PART II

DKFD Food

CHAPTER 5

HOW TO PREPARE FOR AND GET STARTED ON THE DKFD

When Terry and I were getting ready to design our dream home . . . well, let me back up, when *I* was getting ready to design our dream home, I thought about the kitchen almost more than any other space. Let's be honest, my champagne art wall was definitely my #1 display priority. I wanted the space to be open and inviting, spacious enough so that we could have meals with the entire family and a few of the kids' friends if they were to drop in. Another big priority was to have the primary food storage spaces— the refrigerator and pantry—maximize the visibility of healthy foods and snacks.

What we ended up with was exactly what I envisioned—lots of shelving for glass jars filled with baking ingredients, nuts, and snacks, and a fridge that would house the beautiful crisp veggies and fruit from our garden (and the store). We also designed the refrigerator to have plenty of storage space for prepped food so that, even in a pinch, there's always a healthy option available instead of chips!

As you get ready to start the DKFD, I want you to think about your own dreams (the ones that a dietary change can make possible!) . . . whether it's your ideal body or health status, or a combination of the two, and what this could help you achieve. Maybe you want to lose weight so you'll feel comfortable throwing on a bathing suit to hit the water park with your kids like I recently did (as far as dreams go, I can say from experience *aim higher* . . .), or you're hoping that remodeling your metabolism will help you get off cholesterol or type 2 diabetes medication. Or perhaps you're approaching a big birthday and you are thinking, "Whoa, I better turn this ship around before it's too late."

Whatever your dream is, there are steps you can take.

Your pursuit should begin with a remodel of *your* kitchen. Seriously. There is no other space that will be as important to creating your success on this plan. The good thing is that you won't need to hire an architect or contractor to do any kind of work. Although you will probably need to "demo" some of the foods you have now.

After you "remodel" your kitchen, share a snapshot on Instagram and tag us @dubrowketofusiondiet!

Here's the full plan for your DKFD Kitchen Remodel:

Step 1: Demolition of Destructive Foods

Clear your pantry of "factory" carbs, those highly processed foods such as chips, cookies, candy, crackers, sugary cereals, pretzels, white bread, and anything else that might fit in this category. If you're a parent, you might be panicking at this suggestion since most kids love this type of stuff and practically demand that it be available to them. In our house, I try to teach my kids that you can have everything in moderation—I feel like if I make it totally taboo, they'll just go crazy eating crap when they're at friends' houses or out on their own eventually.

That being said, I think when you are first starting a program, it can represent a great moment to review the whole family's diet and point out ways to do better. And you may be surprised to find out your kids can be of great support to you when you explain what you're doing and why you're doing it.

One way to keep these foods in the house without sabotaging yourself is to simply find a separate space for them—a closet or garage or anywhere where they won't be super easy to grab when you're having a snack attack. You can also start to phase in healthy snacks like hard-boiled eggs and nuts and olives; kids are way more inclined to try these foods if you're setting them an example.

As for your fridge: It's time to get rid of fruit juices, sodas, sugary dairy—yogurt, low-fat milk, any kind of flavored or sweetened milk, sweetened nondairy milks—sweetened salad dressings, pudding or Jell-O cups, and condiments containing added sugar, such as ketchup, sweet relish, honey-mustard, barbecue sauce, and teriyaki sauce.

I know this sounds a little extreme and kind of depressing, but this isn't a lifelong sentence of no sweetness ever again—you are simply working to reset your metabolism and eventually you'll be able to reintroduce certain favorites. The goal is to minimize (or even erase) temptations that might derail your progress. And when I say "might," I mean will, because who are we kidding? No one can resist a few handfuls of tortilla chips or a couple of cookies when they're hungry and just getting home!

Minimizing household temptations will also help with reprogramming your palate—when you remove anything that's hypersweet, you give your taste buds a chance to appreciate the natural sweetness found in certain vegetables and herbs; flavors you may not pick up if you're eating a lot of foods containing refined sugars and flours.

And don't forget your freezer—the ice cream, ice cream bars, and popsicles; the frozen glazed chicken entrées; the fruit pies, etc.—give them to your friends (the ones you secretly don't like . . . just kidding, sort of), or have a See Ya Later Sweets party.

Step 2: Pick Out Your New Food "Furniture"

Eating how you want to eat for your health does not happen by accident—you've got to have the right foods (we'll get to these in the Food Lists in Chapter 5) and they have to be right where you can see them. This is why you want to have as many clear containers as possible. Get a few glass containers for your fridge so you can keep some olives, hard-boiled eggs, cut celery, and other snackable veggies right in front. You can also get glass jars for your pantry or countertop; these can be filled with nourishing nuts such as macadamia, walnuts, pecans, and Brazil nuts, or seeds such as pumpkin, hemp, and sesame that you can use to top Greek yogurt, cottage cheese, or a salad.

Keep in mind that you don't have to go out and buy a bunch of new containers, unless of course you want to . . . I know I always enjoy a good excuse for shopping. What you can do instead is repurpose peanut butter, pickle, condiment, or any other type of glass jars as food storage containers. Just be sure to completely clean the inside of the containers, and soak them in hot water if you want to remove the exterior labels.

You will also want to make sure you have plenty of to-go containers so you can pack up any leftover goodies from your new favorite restaurant Chez Moi (i.e., your own home kitchen). The best part of this restaurant is it's very close by and you can show up in your slippers and sweats . . . and the worst part is, well, probably that there's no dishwasher on staff! But the food is incredible (I can't wait for you to try some of the recipes starting on page 103).

Plating is important, too. Bigger plates tend to mean bigger portions, or they may make perfectly filling portions seem small and trick your mind into thinking you haven't had enough food. On the DKFD, we don't want you to be super strict about portions—no need to get a food scale or anything crazy like that. But since we do want you to avoid the problem of overnutrition, it will be helpful to pay more attention to how much you eat. As an experiment, try eating a few meals off of smaller plates, say 9-inch instead of the 12-inch standard size. You might end up going back for seconds, and that's fine. Take your time and savor your meal and see if you notice any difference in how you feel fullness-wise. Another great thing about Chez Moi is that *you* control the portion sizes, whereas most restaurants will actually give you more food than you need to fill up.

Step 3: Add Some Color to Your Spice Selection

If you cook at home a lot already, you probably have an established spice drawer filled with your favorites. While I'm not suggesting you dump these, unless your favorite "spice" is a spoonful of sugar, I do want to encourage you to move in some new spice options. Even upgrading your salt and pepper can make a difference:

* If you've traditionally used iodized salt, try coarse kosher salt for saltiness with a bit more texture, or pick up some Himalayan pink salt or Celtic salt, both of which have more added minerals than traditional salt.
* If you don't already use a pepper grinder, get one for at-home use. Enjoying freshly ground pepper on your salads or soups or main meals doesn't have to be something that only

happens at restaurants—you can make it gourmet with a simple grinder and whole black peppercorns. Seriously, so good!

You'll also find a lot of fantastic spices in our recipes. Spices such as ground ancho chile pepper, mustard powder, chipotle chile powder, dried dill and parsley, and onion and garlic powders are all great for adding so much flavor.

Step 4: Treat Yourself to Some New Tools

In Chapter 6, you'll find over fifty recipes to try. Before you get cooking, I suggest you pick up a few of these useful kitchen tools that we love to have around. Even though I don't cook often, I *loooove* all things surrounding cooking—cooking shows, cookbooks, and cooking utensils—and of course, eating!

You don't need all of these tools to be able to make the DKFD recipes, but they can make preparing some of our favorites a bit easier and even add a little fun! No need to break the bank and seek out the best of all time—just look for tools that seem sturdy enough to last. You can also check stores like Marshalls and Home-Goods for great deals on kitchen tools.

Rimmed baking sheet: When you want to prep meats and veggies (which you'll be doing a lot of on this diet!), a rimmed baking sheet beats a cookie sheet every time. Rimmed baking sheets have a metal "roll" all the way around the perimeter of the pan (so you might see them also described as "jelly-roll pans"), which makes them good for cooking foods that have juices—no spills!

Salad spinner: If you already make salads at home, you probably have one of these simple tools that is a colander and a vegetable dryer in one. Toss in a whole lot of veggies, give them a really good rinse and spin, and you're ready to go. You can also do this ahead of time and then just put it all back in the fridge until you're ready to make your meal. The salad spinner is also one of my secrets to getting liquid out of potatoes when I make latkes every year for Chanukah! It's more multipurpose than you think.

Spiralizer: Spiralizers can make veggies fun by turning them into curly or wide noodles. My personal favorite noodle is pappardelle-style zoodles (made from zucchini): It's a wide flat zoodle that is really nice looking and feels substantial! The only problem is that some spiralizers can make kind of wimpy noodles so you want to look for the best-reviewed one you can afford and give it a try.

Mandoline: A mandoline is a super-sharp, amazing tool for cutting vegetables into uniform slices. Watch your fingers— even pro chefs know to use this tool with caution! Note: This is not a great tool for your younger "chefs" for this reason.

Chef's knife: A sharp, standard chef's knife is essential. Seriously, if you're trying to cut food for your meals with a small steak knife or something like that, you owe it to yourself to get a decent chef's knife. You can find one for $50 or less, but be open to spending a little more if you can.

Meat mallet: Pounding out chicken breasts or certain cuts of beef with a meat mallet can help them cook evenly and will tenderize meats that may be a bit tough to chew. Plus, if you've had a stressful day, you can take it out on those chicken breasts you're going to make for dinner.

Cutting board: Having a good cutting board is sort of a no-brainer. It gives you a nice flat surface on which to cut ingredients that's not your countertop . . . which may not be all that clean even if it looks like it is. We love bamboo cutting boards; they look great and are super durable. You can use these as the surface for pounding any kind of poultry or meat; just line with plastic wrap first. Cutting boards can also double as kitchen counter-top accessories; there are so many great ones to choose from!

Lint-free kitchen towels: We keep a stack of these cotton towels in a drawer to grab for all sorts of uses in the kitchen. They're good for drying your hands, dishes, pots, pans, vegetables, etc. The lint-free towels are the best since they won't leave any little white bits of residue on things.

Instant-read thermometer: It used to be kind of a pain to check the temperature of foods, but an instant-read thermometer can make it less annoying. And you can find one online for less than $50. Look for one that is waterproof!

Now that you know how to remodel your kitchen to set you up for success, here are shopping lists and tips for each of the three windows of the Dubrow Keto Fusion Diet. Remember, it all starts with a 12-hour fast, followed by an 8-hour period of higher fat intake, with no more than 15 to 20 grams of carbs, and then a 4-hour finish during which you can enjoy a more liberal intake of strategic carbs. Your overall macronutrient goal for this 24-hour period will be to eat 60 to 70 percent of your calories from fat, 20 to 30 percent of your calories from protein, and 40 to 60 grams of low-GI carbs. The Meal Plans we've included in the book in Chapter 7 will allow you to eat according to these guidelines when you follow the DKFD recipes.

While there is no strict calorie rule on this diet, the recommendation is that you eat between 1,500 and 1,800 calories daily if you want to achieve consistent results (do not eat less than 1,200 calories if you are a woman or 1,500 calories if you are a man). Each day included in the Meal Plans will fall within this caloric range. Some men and women who are very active or above average height may need up to 2,000 calories.

Once you've familiarized yourself with the Food Lists, be sure to check out the section called Putting the Food Lists into Practice (page 99) to see how to eat from the lists when you're not following our recipes.

Establishing Your "Before"

Just like you wouldn't appreciate the day as much if there were no night, you won't appreciate your "after" body if you don't document what your "before" looks like. You might be thinking that you know *exactly* how your body feels and looks right now, but in even just a few days it's going to be different (isn't that exciting?) and little details will start to change. For the sake of perspective, we encourage you to snap some front and side images the day before you begin the DKFD. You should also step on the scale and document the number.

And P.S., there is zero shame in whatever your starting point is! Just be proud of yourself for stepping up to try something new and for putting in the effort to get what you want.

And P.P.S., we want to see your success—share your before and afters with @dubrowketofusiondiet on Instagram.

12 Reset

This is where it all begins. Let's say it's the night before you're starting the DKFD. What do you do? You enjoy a meal with a few (or more) sips (or glasses) of wine, champagne, or whatever your indulgence of choice is for the evening . . . I'm not judging. You think a little about what makes you happy in your life, and why it is you want to get healthier by losing the weight you've wanted to get rid of for a long time.

Terry and I are super motivated to stay strong, active, and youthful for as long as possible for our kids.

Our youngest is only eight so we've got to stay on our toes for a long time yet! Being able to keep up with the kids is a huge factor for us, but let's face it: We want to feel as youthful as we look. I'm sure you have your own, equally meaningful and motivating reasons for pursuing better health; and considering these before you dive in is a good way to connect to your purpose and stay motivated during the most challenging parts of the diet.

Now, since your 12-hour Reset begins whenever you finish eating and drinking, and this sets into motion your whole eating schedule, you may want to consider how late into the evening you keep eating, snacking, or drinking anything with calories (obviously you can drink water, and a handful of other things we'll mention on page 78). Here's how your eating schedule could shape up depending on your last meal of the day:

RESET BEGINS	RESET ENDS	RECHARGE BEGINS	RECHARGE ENDS	REFUEL BEGINS	REFUEL ENDS
8 p.m.	8 a.m.	8 a.m.	4 p.m.	4 p.m.	8 p.m.
9 p.m.	9 a.m.	9 a.m.	5 p.m.	5 p.m.	9 p.m.
10 p.m.	10 a.m.	10 a.m.	6 p.m.	6 p.m.	10 p.m.
11 p.m.	11 a.m.	11 a.m.	7 p.m.	7 p.m.	11 p.m.

If you work on an unconventional schedule, you can shift these time windows to reflect your specific sleep-wake schedule.

Since the first window of the DKFD is dedicated to fasting, this means no food or beverages (unless it's a small amount of non-insulin-stimulating, very low-carb calories). When you abstain from eating during these 12 hours, you will kick off an awesome metabolic chain of action that will lead to increased fat burning. Of course, your metabolism is different from mine, which is different from Terry's, and so on, meaning it will take each person a different amount of time to get to a fat-burning state. But generally speaking, metabolic insight suggests that it takes at least 12 hours before the body reaches a need to use stored fat for energy.

Remember, the ultimate goal of this Reset period is to shut down fat storage, which is what happens when insulin is present, and shift your internal system to fat burning instead, which is what happens when insulin is *not* present.

If you're feeling apprehensive about fasting, I can assure you there's nothing to be afraid of. I still remember when Terry talked a ton about fasting and how much he loved it and I pretty quickly started zoning out as I thought it might be one of his extreme ideas, you know, not really my thing. My personal thoughts on the topic were summed up by a simple "Fasting? Hmm. No thank you."

Then I started looking deeper at the details of my own eating schedule. I used to be all about the bagel in the mornings (it's the New Yorker in me!), but it always made me feel heavy, full, and super low-energy. Once I ditched that routine and started having just some water and maybe a powdered supplement drink, like the Primo Beets and Primo Celery we make with our Consult Health line, before going straight into a workout, I noticed I felt so much better. I didn't have that poochy belly fullness that I hate, I had way more energy, and I could really commit to my workouts. Once

I started doing that, I usually wouldn't eat my first meal until around 10, even 11 a.m.

You may have noticed that this sounds quite a bit like a Reset period, and it was—it turns out I was unintentionally fasting for at least 12 hours (this is why I like to refer to myself as the accidental faster). I'm telling you this because it shows you that it doesn't have to be difficult, and in fact it can make you feel good enough that you want to keep doing it on purpose.

Once I was consistently committed to a Reset interval, Terry and I worked together to identify the short list of items that would help make the fasting period of our diet as pleasurable as possible. Here's the short list of what's allowed during the Reset:

* Water: Regular water, sparkling water, ice water, lemon water . . . all good! Go for sparkling water options with no sugar, such as LaCroix. Don't be afraid to get creative with the water you drink, either. I love to create naturally fla-vored varieties for myself by adding a few squeezes of fresh citrus to my water bottle, or even spicing it up a little with cayenne and some lemon juice. Terry adds crushed ice to his water because he says it's more thirst quenching and since satiety receptors (which indicate hunger satisfaction) are temperature sensitive, the colder liquids can make you feel fuller even when you're fasting.

* Coffee: So many people live for their first cup of coffee in the morning, and the thought of having to fast without coffee would likely make them quit immediately. If you're one of those people, you'll be happy to know that coffee is com-pletely fine during the Reset window. What's not fine is any type of coffee drink that's full of added sugars or regular milk. No blended coffee drinks topped with whipped cream and chocolate or caramel sauce. If you are used to drinking

sweet coffee and absolutely can't do without, you can try adding a small amount of stevia or monk fruit sweetener. Ideally you want to adapt to no sweetener to help prevent any increase in sugar cravings, but you can work your way toward that if needed.

* **Tea:** Black, green, oolong, herbal, yerba maté, and unsweetened fruit teas are acceptable while fasting. If you're questioning whether something has sweeteners or added sugar, simply check the label or ask before you order.

* **Heavy cream:** The best thing to add to your coffee or tea during your Reset window is heavy cream. Two tablespoons of heavy cream has under 1 gram of carbohydrate, making it the best choice for fasting. If you need a nondairy option, you can also use nondairy creamer or a small amount of unsweetened almond milk.

* **Bone broth/bouillon:** While "bone broth" has a rather unappetizing ring to it, it can be a great source of quick nourishment to get you through to the Recharge window. This type of broth is similar to a stock but is generally cooked longer to extract collagen from bones (typically from chicken or beef). While we haven't seen any research that supports a lot of the claims made about bone broth, it can provide a decent dose of supportive minerals and serve as a low-calorie and no-carbohydrate way to fill an empty stomach until your fast is over. You can also dissolve one bouillon cube in warm water for a quick burst of flavor and a dose of sodium.

* **Beet supplement:** Beets are one of the best sources of natural nitrates, which when consumed can help increase production of nitric oxide, a molecule that can help relax blood vessels and increase blood flow. We like to try to take advantage of this benefit by drinking a powdered beet supplement in the mornings. We created our own version called

Primo Beets with our Consult Health line, which doesn't have added sugar and is low in calories. I love it because I can't normally do a lot of coffee first thing in the morning, so I drink this for energy instead. You can use any beet supplement of your choice. Just look for one that has no added sugar!

* Celery supplement or greens-based supplement drink: We've worked hard to try to find ways that we can get vitamins and minerals into the hours that we spend fasting (without experiencing any kind of stomach upset that can be caused by multivitamins or triggering the glucose-insulin response). Two of our favorite options are the ones we designed with our team called Primo Celery and Primo Greens. (You might think we're biased because we created these supplements and, well, we are—we love them almost as much as our own children! But we really have gone through dozens of versions to make sure they match up with how we eat and how you're going to eat on this plan.)

I love the celery powder because it's super hydrating, you can have it on an empty stomach without feeling funky, and it helps keep your bowel movements regular. This last one is a major plus especially if the DKFD represents your first foray into a low-carbohydrate type of diet. These types of diets are notorious for contributing to constipation. Drinking plenty of water is key to avoiding this, but celery juice can also provide an essential digestive boost when you need it—or act as a typical part of your keeping-it-regular routine.

The Primo Greens are great, too, and include a greens blend made from a ton of true superfoods, such as wheatgrass, spirulina, matcha tea, blue-green algae, broccoli, kale, chlorella, spinach, and more.

You can drink any kind of powdered celery or greens-based powder of your choice. To make sure they're acceptable during your Reset window, check the nutritional label—no added sugars allowed, and you ideally want them to be under 15 calories. While you don't have to be a calorie counter on this plan, during the fasting period, you don't want to overdo it, even with noncarb calories.

Of course, none of these items except water are required—they are all optional and included only if you find you need something to sip on while fasting. We found that we liked to experiment with different combinations of things to see what made each of us feel our best, and we encourage you to try this as well. This ends up meaning that you skip coffee on some days after you find that a beets-based drink is all you need for morning energy. Or maybe you'll discover a new type of tea that tastes like such a treat that you can't wait to get up and out of bed to enjoy it. Don't be afraid to splurge a little on whatever it is you find you like best during the fasting window. Try that exotic coffee blend or order a special Japanese tea; you deserve it!

If you find you're having a hard time hitting the 12-hour mark, here are a few strategies to try:

* **Extend your fast.** This might sound counterintuitive, but since you are in a sort of self-experimentation mode, you want to be open to trying modifications that could make a difference, and extending your fast might be the shift that makes it more successful for you. So, here's how you would extend it: If you ate your last bit of food around 8 p.m., try going until 10 a.m. the next day before consuming anything other than what's on the short list (making it a 14-hour fast). In this case, whatever you ate before bed will be better di-

gested before you go to sleep and this could make a difference in how you feel hungerwise in the morning.

* Increase your sodium intake. Try some Himalayan pink salt to
increase your mineral intake or heat up some bone broth
and drink a cup to see if that gets you through any rough
patches.

* Talk yourself through it. A 12-hour fast is very doable, especially
if you tell yourself it is. Sometimes the discomfort we experience around adopting something new is more a reaction
to the newness itself than anything else. We become so ad-
dicted to the patterns that shape our lives, and these patterns definitely include when and what we eat, even how we
eat. We want to use that one glass bowl that's really good for
big pasta dishes, or those specific plates for pizza night, even
though we probably have plenty of other options that would
work. You are making a change to how you eat; you know
how to do it, and you know you can do it. Remind yourself
of this when you experience any challenging moments.

Once you've completed the Reset window, you're ready to jump
into Recharge. This will be eight hours of time during which you
will want to eat a diet higher in selective fats and very low in carbohydrates.

8 Recharge

When you reach this part of your day (or night, if that's how your
schedule works), we want you to think about eating with purpose.
Of course, you'll be hungry, so part of that purpose will be simply
to satisfy that appetite you've worked up through your dedication
to fasting. But your bigger purpose will be to eat in a way that will

extend the metabolic effects of your fast without requiring you to extend the actual fast.

You accomplish this by eating certain high-fat foods (see list on page 85) and consuming no more than 15 grams of carbohydrates. This keto-ish way of eating will be the key to not activating the fat-storage cycle kicked off by a sudden introduction of a high-carb meal. Keto will keep a good thing going.

Since this isn't a pure keto diet, you likely won't go into a full ketotic state where you're burning ketones 24/7, and that's totally fine. Because you know what else you won't have to go into—the dreaded "keto flu." Okay, the keto flu isn't really affiliated with any type of influenza, but it has been known to make people feel pretty lousy by contributing to symptoms such as nausea, headaches, and overall increased tiredness.

Ask Dr. Dubrow: "Should I Be Testing for Ketones?"

You may have heard that some people on ketogenic diets like to test for the presence of ketones, something that can be done by checking blood, breath, or urine. Since the Dubrow Keto Fusion Diet is a lower ketone producer, thanks to the inclusion of low-glycemic carbs, it's not necessary or even worth the time and effort to test. We do encourage you, however, to "test" your metabolic results by paying attention to how you feel. I know that for me there are unquestionable, noticeable benefits, including better focus, better sleep, and better ability to handle stress, all of which improve my job performance (people don't really like a sleepy surgeon) and help me enjoy time with my family more. As you adapt to the diet, watch for these improvements, which occur as a result of better glucose control, intermittent introduction of ketones, and increased intake of high-nutrient foods.

It's a bit of mystery why some people develop keto flu symptoms, but it could be a result of the underlying metabolic transition being initiated by the dramatic increase in fat and decrease in carbohydrates. This transition lowers blood sugar, leading to less insulin being present, which can by itself lead to greater fluids and electrolytes being excreted from the body. When this happens, dehydration and electrolyte imbalances can develop and lead to issues such as headaches and muscle cramps.

We've included strategic carbs in the DKFD to eliminate such a dramatic drop in carbohydrate consumption, minimizing the chance of unpleasant symptoms such as these. It is possible, however, that if your "before" diet was extremely high in processed carbs, the DKFD as your "after" diet may produce some adjustment side effects.

To further minimize the chance of these occurring, follow these tips:

1. **Be sure to eat enough low-GI carbs!** These shouldn't be considered optional. Eating plenty of filling, nutrient-packed, nonstarchy veggies and fresh herbs from the Food List, and approved grains and resistant starch desserts during the Refuel window will be critical in preventing unpleasant symptoms.

2. **Drink water with a water chaser.** When you change your diet, you are essentially introducing a new metabolic workout to your cells, one that will "exercise" potentially out-of-shape chemical interactions and fuel-use systems. Drinking plenty of water can help your cells adapt better to new demands. It can also help alleviate headaches and muscle cramps that some people experience when they modify their carbohydrate intake. Aim to drink about 6 to 8 glasses of water a day.

3. **Get salty.** Increased electrolyte loss means reduced levels of sodium, magnesium, and potassium, which control electrical impulses in the body that impact muscle contractions, fluid levels, heart rhythm, blood pressure, and more. If you do notice any kind of funky, flu-like feelings coming on, aim to get a little more of these three electrolytes into your diet. Add extra salt to your dishes (or drink some bone broth), and eat extra dark leafy greens, avocado, spinach, and black beans. You're probably not used to having someone suggest adding salt to your food, but because we are pretty much wiping out all processed foods from your diet, you'll have a bit more room to add some quality salts for flavor and electrolyte balance. If you have high blood pressure or have been advised to follow a low-sodium diet, check with your physician before making adjustments to your salt use.

With these tips in mind, it's time for you to go shopping! Use the following Food List to shop for the best of everything to eat during the Recharge window. Remember that you'll want to aim for 15 to 20 grams of carbs during the 8 hours of this window.

Recharge Food List

The first five categories in this list include foods that have no carbs or low-enough carbs that you don't need to worry about keeping track of them. In most cases, we've still included a suggested portion size. This doesn't mean that's all you can eat of these foods, but it does provide you a sense of how to measure them. The later categories, starting with nuts, will include the carbohydrate grams and you can use this information to help you reach 15 to 20 grams per day during the Recharge window (you'll see dairy appear in both categories as some dairy-based foods have more carbohydrates than others). A few additional notes on this list:

* In the categories of foods with very low to no carbs (most fats and/or proteins), the foods have been sorted by percentage of calories from fat, highest to lowest. We have organized them this way to help you get a sense of where you might find foods highest in nutrient-dense fat. This isn't to say you will always need to prioritize those foods at the top of the list, but if you feel you need additional calories or extra-satiating foods, that's where you will want to pick from. P.S. Note that it's the highest percentage of calories from fat, not the highest in fat!

* The carbohydrate grams have been rounded to the nearest whole number. This is to make it a bit easier to add things up.

* You don't have to be militant in portion control or carbohydrate counting, unless you want to. We don't count carbs because we've been eating a low-carb diet for so long that it's sort of second nature. You can use the carbohydrate grams in the Food List as a tool for establishing greater understanding. But once you "get it," you won't have to track anything—you'll just know how to eat for your best results.

* If you haven't tried it, now's the time! If you see anything listed that you haven't tried, be adventurous and get those goodies on your plate. You might even discover your next favorite food!

Of course, do not miss the DKFD recipes starting on page 103. These have been created exclusively for the program in this book and feature some truly outstanding dishes.

OILS (1 TABLESPOON)

Sorted by percentage of calories from fat, highest to lowest.

MCT oil	avocado oil
olive oil	grapeseed oil

walnut oil

coconut oil

almond oil

DAIRY

Sorted by percentage of calories from fat, highest to lowest.

ghee (1 tablespoon)

grass-fed butter (1 tablespoon)

heavy (whipping) cream
(2 tablespoons)

MEATS / FISH / POULTRY / SEAFOOD / EGGS (4 TO 6 OUNCES, UNLESS OTHERWISE NOTED)

Sorted by percentage of calories from fat, highest to lowest.

pancetta (1 ounce)

liver pâté (¼ cup)

pork, spare ribs

pork, shoulder

eggs, chicken or duck (2 or 3)

lamb, loin

pork, bacon, uncured and nitrate-free (4 slices)

beef, rib eye

lamb, chops

shad

beef, New York strip steak

beef, grass-fed, lean ground (½ pound)

anchovies, canned in oil

salmon, wild-caught

beef, top sirloin steak

bison, grass-fed, ground (½ pound)

duck

beef, skirt steak

chicken, dark meat

turkey, dark meat

sea bass

bone broth (1 cup)

SPICES

coriander

cumin

cayenne pepper

basil

turmeric

black pepper

chile pepper

cinnamon

cloves

dill

ginger

Himalayan pink salt

lemon pepper	rosemary
mustard seeds or powder	sage
oregano	Spike (super-tasty blend of spices)
parsley	thyme
peppermint	

CONDIMENTS / DRESSING INGREDIENTS (1 TABLESPOON)

Sorted by percentage of calories from fat, highest to lowest.

avocado oil mayonnaise without added sugars	wasabi
	sriracha
Duke's mayonnaise	rice vinegar
Japanese Kewpie mayo	white wine vinegar
horseradish	apple cider vinegar
soy sauce	fish sauce
tamari	lemon juice

NUTS (PORTION = ABOUT 2 GRAMS CARBS)

Sorted by percentage of calories from fat, highest to lowest.

pecans (10 halves)	coconut, shredded (¼ cup)
Brazil nuts (3 nuts)	hazelnuts (10 nuts)
macadamia nuts (6 nuts)	pine nuts (2 tablespoons)
walnuts (7 halves)	almonds (10 nuts)

NUT AND SEED BUTTERS (1 TABLESPOON = ABOUT 3 GRAMS CARBS)

Sorted by percentage of calories from fat, highest to lowest.

macadamia nut butter (lowest in carbs)	tahini
	almond butter
pecan butter	
walnut butter	

SEEDS / SNACKS (PORTION = ABOUT 2 GRAMS CARBS)

Sorted by percentage of calories from fat, highest to lowest.

hemp (2 tablespoons)

pumpkin (½ ounce/about 70 seeds)

sesame (1 tablespoon)

flaxseed, ground (1 tablespoon)

beef jerky, no sugar added (1 ounce)

chia (1 teaspoon)

pickles, no sugar added (1 medium)

OTHER GOOD FATS (PORTION = ABOUT 2 GRAMS CARBS)

Sorted by percentage of calories from fat, highest to lowest.

coconut cream (2 tablespoons)

olives, pitted: black, green, Kalamata (½ cup)

Dairy-Free Like Me? Try These!

We have plenty of dairy in the house for Terry and the kids, but I cannot do dairy, so I also make sure we always have plenty of delicious nondairy options stocked in the pantry and fridge. Here are some of my favorites:

FOOD	AMOUNT	CARBOHYDRATE (G)
Ripple Half and Half (original)	2 tablespoons	0
coconut cream (unsweetened)	2 tablespoons	0
coconut milk	1 cup	1
Ripple pea milk (unsweetened original)	1 cup	1
Lactaid whole milk	½ cup	7

DAIRY		
FOOD	AMOUNT	CARBOHYDRATE (G)
mozzarella, whole-milk	¾ cup shredded; 3 slices	2
parmesan	½ cup	2

FOOD	AMOUNT	CARBOHYDRATE (G)
cottage cheese, whole-milk	1/2 cup	3
Greek yogurt, whole-milk	1/2 cup	5

FRUITS (THAT ACT LIKE VEGGIES)

FOOD	AMOUNT	CARBOHYDRATE (G)
avocado	1/2	6
tomato, chopped	1/2 cup	3

VEGETABLES

FOOD	AMOUNT	CARBOHYDRATE (G)
chives, chopped	1 tablespoon	0
arugula	3/4 cup	0
ginger, minced	1 tablespoon	0
watercress	1 cup	0
cilantro	1 cup	1
garlic	1 clove	1
seaweed	10 sheets	1
onion, thinly sliced	5 slices	1
jalapeño, diced	1 pepper	1
endive, chopped	1 cup	1
bok choy, shredded	1/2 cup	2
alfalfa sprouts	4 ounces	2
bamboo shoots, sliced	1/2 cup	2
green onion, chopped	1/4 cup	2
mustard greens, chopped	1 cup	3
celery	2 stalks	3
broccoli, chopped	1/2 cup	3
asparagus	5 spears	3

FOOD	AMOUNT	CARBOHYDRATE (G)
fennel, sliced	$1/2$ cup	3
Chinese broccoli, chopped	1 cup	3
pattypan squash, sliced	$1/2$ cup	3
lettuce, all varieties	2 cups	3
shallots, chopped	2 tablespoons	3
mushrooms, sliced	1 cup	3
green beans, cut into $1/2$-inch pieces	$1/2$ cup	4
grape leaves	8 leaves	4
green bell pepper, sliced	1 cup	4
eggplant, cubed	$1/2$ cup	4
cauliflower, chopped	$1/2$ cup	5
dandelion greens	1 cup	5
bean sprouts	1 cup	5
snow peas/green peas	$1/2$ cup	6
zucchini	1 medium	6
kale, chopped	1 cup	6
brussels sprouts	6 sprouts	6
sauerkraut	1 cup	6
spinach	1 cup	7
artichokes	$1/2$ artichoke	7
parsley, chopped	$1/2$ cup	7
okra	1 cup	7
chard, all varieties, chopped	1 cup	7
cucumber	1 medium	7
leeks, sliced	$1/2$ cup	6
chile peppers	2 peppers	8
cabbage, all types, shredded	1 cup	8
collard greens, chopped	1 cup	11

SWEETENERS (1 TEASPOON)
stevia   monk fruit

BAKING INGREDIENTS		
FOOD	AMOUNT	CARBOHYDRATE (G)
almond flour	2 tablespoons	5
arrowroot powder	$1/2$ tablespoon	4

4 Refuel

Once you've reached the Refuel window, you've dedicated 20 hours of time to metabolic reconstruction—and that's no small feat. (You don't need to tell anyone that you might have spent 7 or 8 of those hours sleeping . . . your body does a lot of work during that time, so it still counts!) The final 4 hours of the DKFD day will be about carrying forward your commitment to eating nutrient-rich fats and adding to that some low-glycemic carbs. These strategically selected carbs will help prevent carb withdrawal and provide plenty of vitamins and minerals that you would miss out on if you were following a pure keto diet.

You've already discovered that low-GI carbs will help keep your glucose response relatively slow, preventing any excessive insulin response. You might also be interested in knowing that there are a few extra steps you can take to ensure that the glycemic index of your meals stays low:

1. **Don't overcook your carbs.** The more refined, processed, or cooked a carbohydrate is, the greater the glucose response. This is because foods in these lesser forms enter the digestive system ready to be used immediately and demand a

sudden and significant increase in insulin. On the flip side, when a carb is kept intact, that is, eaten with fiber, or when it's more al dente, there's greater digestive effort required. More work means slower processing and a slower, measured insulin response. To prevent an increase in a carbohydrate's glycemic index, avoid overcooking it. This includes everything from vegetables to pasta.

2. **Avoid overripe fruits.** Overripe fruits have a higher concentration of sugars and therefore deliver a more concentrated dose of glucose. Eat fruits just as they ripen or even when they are slightly underripe.

3. **Use acidic dressings.** Adding something acidic such as a dressing made with vinegar or lemon to any carb-containing meal can help slow the conversion of carbohydrate molecules into glucose.

4. **Pair carbs with fat.** Similar to adding an acidic food, pairing carbs with fat can help slow carb conversion and bring the speed of the entire digestive process down, which means you stay fuller longer.

Be sure to also include resistant starches in your diet. These stand-alone carbs essentially avoid the standard digestive process, which is why I like to call them invisible carbs. Of course, your body processes them so they're not actually invisible, but instead of being metabolized like other types of carbohydrates, they actually get broken down by the good bacteria in your gut.

I'm feeling satisfied because I am not eating endless amounts of sugar and empty carbs. My meals last and make me feel great for longer periods of time!

—KELLY BERLIN

Some of the carbs that are already included in the Refuel Food List because they're low-glycemic are also resistant starches. These are foods such as lentils and white beans, and certain grains such as barley. Other resistant starches that we've added include raw green banana flour and cooked then cooled rice. Rice that's been cooked then cooled has been estimated to have 50 to 60 percent fewer calories than cooked rice. I'm not a chemist, so I'm not exactly sure how this happens, but it seems that cooling a cooked starch helps increase its resistant starch content, which in turn makes it have less of an effect on glucose response.

To take advantage of this loophole in carbohydrate chemistry, you can simply cook foods such as rice and beans and then put them in the fridge overnight or for 24 hours, and then reheat and eat. Pro tip: Reheating doesn't lower the resistant starch.

Refuel Food List

These foods can be added to what was included on the previous Food Lists. Since your total low-GI carb intake for the day should be no more than 50 to 60 grams, be sure to carry forward whatever you ate in the Recharge window and include that in your total. Also, be sure to continue to eat foods higher in fat, which were featured on the previous list.

MEATS / FISH / POULTRY / SEAFOOD / EGGS (4 TO 6 OUNCES, UNLESS OTHERWISE NOTED)

sardines, canned in oil (1 can)	oysters (6 to 12)
beef tenderloin	chicken, white meat
trout, steelhead	mussels (1 pound, in shells)
tuna, canned in oil (1 5-ounce can)	halibut
salmon, canned (1 5-ounce can)	crab
swordfish	clams (1 pound, in shells)
pork tenderloin	turkey, white meat

mahimahi   tuna: ahi, bluefin, yellowfin

cod

DAIRY

FOOD	AMOUNT	CARBOHYDRATE (G)
ricotta, whole milk	$^1/_2$ cup	6
whole milk	$^1/_2$ cup	6

VEGETABLES

FOOD	AMOUNT	CARBOHYDRATE (G)
endive	1 head	2
radishes, sliced	1 cup	3
shallots	1 shallot	7
cucumber	1 medium	7
red bell pepper	1 pepper	8
yellow bell pepper	1 pepper	8
spaghetti squash, cubed	1 cup	10
jicama, sliced	1 cup	11
carrots, chopped (raw or steamed)	1 cup	12
water chestnuts	1 cup	17
acorn squash, cubed	1 cup	20
butternut squash, cubed	1 cup	22

FRUITS

FOOD	AMOUNT	CARBOHYDRATE (G)
coconut, raw, shredded	$^1/_2$ cup	6
limes	1 fruit	7
plums	1 fruit	8
lemons	1 fruit	8
blackberries	1 cup	14

FOOD	AMOUNT	CARBOHYDRATE (G)
raspberries	1 cup	15
apples, sliced	1 cup	16
peaches	1 fruit	17
oranges	1 fruit	18
tart cherries	1 cup	19
strawberries	1 cup	20
blueberries	1 cup	21
grapefruit, sliced	1 cup	25
pears	1 fruit	27

RESISTANT STARCHES

FOOD	AMOUNT	CARBOHYDRATE (G)
"Invisible Rice" (page 177)	$^1/_2$ cup	11*
green banana flour, uncooked	2 tablespoons	13
whole wheat or multigrain bread	1 slice	14
bulgur	$^1/_2$ cup	17
sweet potato, cubed	$^1/_2$ cup	19
lima beans	$^1/_2$ cup	20
kidney beans	$^1/_2$ cup	20
lentils	$^1/_2$ cup	20
quinoa	$^1/_2$ cup	20
black beans	$^1/_2$ cup	21
barley	$^1/_2$ cup	22
chickpeas	$^1/_2$ cup	23
pinto beans	$^1/_2$ cup	23
brown rice	$^1/_2$ cup	23
oats, rolled	$^1/_2$ cup	27

*Based on research that estimates cooking and cooling rice lowers calories by 50 percent.

CONDIMENTS/DRESSING INGREDIENTS		
FOOD	AMOUNT	CARBOHYDRATE (G)
balsamic vinegar	1 tablespoon	3

SWEETENERS		
FOOD	AMOUNT	CARBOHYDRATE (G)
erythritol	1 teaspoon	4

ALCOHOL (MEN: 1 OR 2 DRINKS PER NIGHT; WOMEN: 1 DRINK PER NIGHT)	
brut champagne (Heather's favorite!)	vodka
	tequila
brandy	whisky
gin	

Alcohol on the DKFD

Heather and I have always been open about our love for alcohol, whether it's a tasty tequila cocktail (for me) or a bubbly glass of brut champagne (for her). These are definitely indulgences we allow ourselves to enjoy. Like we've said, you don't need to cut out *every single thing* you love, but moderation is critical.

Luckily for all the bubbly lovers out there, alcohol is something you can enjoy as well while following the program. There are, however, some guidelines to keep in mind.

During the first three weeks, consider limiting your alcohol intake to just your cheat day. Yes, this means drinking only once a week, but hear me out. When you first begin the DKFD, you are eating to reconstruct your metabolism and specifically to train your cells to shift toward efficient fat burning.

When you drink alcohol, even varieties that are low in sugar (i.e., carbs), your system prioritizes metabolizing this substance over other sources of metabolic fuel. In this instance, utilization of fatty acids can get put on hold. We don't want that to happen.

Beyond the first three weeks, you can consider incorporating one drink a night for women and one or two drinks per night for men. This is by no means a dietary requirement or recommendation even, but moderate alcohol intake has been shown to have benefits. One study, led by Associate Professor of Epidemiology at Columbia University Katherine M. Keyes, found that moderate and occasional drinkers may be less likely to die prematurely than people who abstain from alcohol entirely. Other research has shown potential heart-related benefits of alcohol, introduced by its ability to prevent plaque buildup in the arteries.

When you do drink, it's smart to avoid overdoing it, no matter where you are in the diet (or whether you're dieting at all, for that matter). Binge drinking, defined as more than four or five drinks within about two hours at least one day a month, is bad news for your body and long-term health. According to the American Addiction Center, recurrent binge drinking has been linked to increased risk for

* the development of damage to the liver, such as cirrhosis
* numerous forms of cancer
* renal issues
* menstrual issues in women and impotence in men
* cardiovascular disorders, such as high blood pressure, heart attack, stroke
* neurological issues, including nerve pain, movement disorders, and dementia
* cognitive issues, such as problems with memory, attention, and problem-solving
* mental health issues, such as anxiety, depression, bipolar disorder, and psychotic disorders

Given these risks, you can see clearly why moderation is paramount, but that doesn't mean you can't still enjoy the party (I mean, we have a champagne art wall!). Indulge smartly by drinking just one or two drinks per night. For the purposes of weight loss and weight maintenance while following the DKFD, it's best to avoid high-sugar and high-carb alcoholic beverages such as sweet blended drinks or craft beers (see the better alcohol choices on page 97).

It should be noted that you may find that you're more sensitive to alcohol while following this diet. Since you will likely have less available glucose, alcohol will be metabolized quickly, and you may experience the feeling of it "going straight to your head"—because it is. This shouldn't necessarily be cause for concern, but it is something to which you should pay attention.

Putting the Food Lists into Practice

In the next two chapters, you'll find recipes and meal plans, both of which Terry and I want to encourage you to use as much as possible as you get started with the DKFD. But we also want you to think of these a little bit like culinary "crutches"—meaning they'll be perfect to help you get around when you first get started, but ultimately you'll want to learn to walk on your own by using the Food Lists to craft and create your own meals. This is how you will ensure the best results long-term.

While doing so should not be difficult, it will take time to get into a groove with a new way of eating. I know it took me a little while to adjust to incorporating more fat in my diet, but I seriously love eating this way so much now!

I want to share some tips with you in terms of how to approach eating from the Food Lists during each window of the DKFD.

Reset: Obviously the easiest in terms of what you can consume since the list of approved items is pretty short! Since you'll be fasting, you'll want to stick to what's on the list on pages 78–81.

Recharge: The goal here is to pick a quality protein to pair with some nutrient-rich fats and enjoy with a serving or two of low-GI veggies. You will just want to make sure that you're eating carbs from the Food List on pages 85–92 and that your carbohydrate intake doesn't go over 20 grams. Look for opportunities to add healthy fats such as avocado, nuts, or olives.

During this 8-hour window, you can eat two smaller meals—like a late breakfast plus a late lunch, or you can enjoy a fat-enriched coffee or tea and a bigger meal at lunch. Another option is to enjoy a coffee + lunch + a delicious snack (hard-boiled or deviled eggs are great; nut butters with celery, roasted nuts, cheese, olives, salami . . . all good snack foods!). Feel free to experiment to find what works best for you, and switch it up whenever you find you're more or less hungry.

Refuel: The basic formula is pretty similar here to the Recharge window—quality protein, nutrient-rich fats, and low-GI veggies—but you can bump up the veggie quantity and be sure to add in a resistant starch from the list. These include foods such as barley, quinoa, lentils, black beans, chickpeas, etc. (you can see the full list beginning on page 94).

This diet is making me pay closer attention to what I'm fueling my body with. I pay attention to portion sizes and listen to my body when I'm beginning to get full. I don't see myself ever going back to eating like I used to.

—BRITTANY BEST

And there you have it—what I would call the ABCs of eating on the DKFD. Here's an example of how this could look in practice:

12-hour Reset

Two glasses of cold water

One serving of Primo Celery (drink in water)

8-hour Recharge

LATE BREAKFAST: EGG SCRAMBLE WITH AVOCADO

(If you need to make this to-go, you can prep your eggs by soft- or hard-boiling them to create more of a savory breakfast egg salad.)

INGREDIENT	QUANTITY
eggs	2
avocado	$1/3$ avocado
bacon	2 slices
grass-fed butter (or ghee)	$1/2$ tablespoon
baby bella mushrooms, sliced	$1/3$ cup
green bell pepper, sliced	$1/3$ cup

LATE LUNCH: BEEF WITH CAULIFLOWER RICE

INGREDIENT	QUANTITY
grass-fed lean ground beef	5 ounces
garlic	1 clove
cauliflower, medium head	$1/4$ head
avocado	$2/3$ avocado
cherry tomatoes	4 tomatoes
coconut oil	1 tablespoon

DINNER: SALMON WITH GRILLED EGGPLANT

INGREDIENT	QUANTITY
wild salmon	5 ounces
olive oil	$1/2$ tablespoon
lemon juice	1 tablespoon
soy sauce, reduced-sodium	$1/2$ tablespoon
fresh ginger, grated	1 teaspoon
garlic	2 cloves
baby bella mushrooms	$1/3$ cup
coconut oil	1 tablespoon
eggplant	$1/3$ eggplant
pistachios, no salt	1 tablespoon

CHAPTER 6

THE DKFD RECIPES

Welcome to the Dubrow Keto Fusion Diet recipes! There are so many incredible-tasting snacks, sides, and entrées for you to try here. We brought in our amazing chef C. Amanda Jackson to help create outstanding flavor with foods that match the diet. (She's also shared some notes and tips before each recipe, so be sure to read these.) Dig in, and let us know what you love!

RECHARGE RECIPES (8-HOUR WINDOW)

TASTY MORNING COFFEES

SATISFYING SNACKS

Killer Kale Chips (page 117)

Deviled Eggs, 3 Ways (page 118)

Plain

Bacon & Parmesan

Smoked Salmon & Dill

Loaded Celery Sticks (page 120)

BREAKFAST / BRUNCH

Fat Bomb Burger Sliders with Bacon-Wrapped Onion Rings (page 121)

Breakfast Salad with Ranch Dressing (page 123)

Cast-Iron Skillet Frittata (page 125)

Parmesan & Dill Blinis with Smoked Salmon (page 126)

Bacon-Wrapped Breakfast Burgers (page 127)

Cauliflower Bacon Hash with Soft-Boiled Eggs (page 129)

LUNCH / LATE LUNCH / EARLY DINNER

Arugula Salad with Crispy Pan-Roasted Salmon (page 131)

Spinach Salad with Pan-Roasted Lamb Chops (page 133)

Grilled Spatchcock Chicken & Cauliflower Stuffing (page 135)

Southern-Style Shrimp & Cauliflower "Grits" (page 137)

Crispy Chicken Wings with Spicy Mustard Greens (page 139)

Bok Choy Salad with Pan-Seared Tofu (page 141)

Salmon & Avocado Poke with Green "Noodle" Salad (page 143)

Roasted Garlic Butter Steak Bites with Italian Mustard Greens (page 145)

BROTH / DRESSINGS

Keto Bone Broth (page 147)

Ketchup (page 148)

REFUEL RECIPES (4-HOUR WINDOW)

SATISFYING SNACKS

DINNERS

PERFECTLY PAN-ROASTED PROTEINS

Rib Eyes (page 182)

Chicken Breasts (page 183)

Lamb Chops (page 184)

Salmon (page 185)

BUTTERS / SAUCES / SMASHES

Avocado Butter (page 186)

Cajun Butter (page 187)

Caramelized Onion & Herb Butter (page 188)

Anchovy & Herb Butter (page 189)

Olive & Herb Butter (page 190)

Bacon, Parmesan & Herb Butter (page 191)

Hollandaise (page 192)

Avocado & Basil Smash (page 193)

Orange & Dill Infused Ghee (page 194)

Can we talk recipes? The Cauliflower Bacon Hash, Pan-Roasted Lamb Chops, and Crispy Chicken Wings are my favorites. I find it hard to believe I can eat this well and still lose weight and feel amazing—I'm loving this way of living!

—ANDREA CHANG

Eat Your Best Even When You're Busy

You can stick to the plan even during busy weeks by following these tips and picking from the list of recipes that follow:

* Make vinaigrettes ahead of time so you can prep a salad and already have dressings at the ready.
* Pick from any of the pan-roasted proteins, as these are interchangeable and pair well with quick and simple sautéed veggies (select your favorites from the food list).
* Keep your pantry stocked with grains such as barley and quinoa, and always grab a head of cauliflower when you're at the store since there are so many great ways to prepare this cruciferous vegetable. Double the recipe for cauliflower or barley fried rice or quinoa pilaf and you'll find you will go through it quickly on busy weeknights!
* Use a grocery delivery service. There are many services that offer grocery delivery for a small fee. When you feel a whole lot of life piling on, sign up for one of these to help ensure you have the foods you need to stay on track. Then, just cancel the service when things settle down.

Some of the other recipes you'll want to make when you're busy include Salmon & Avocado Poke with Green "Noodle" Salad; Arugula Salad with Crispy Pan-Roasted Salmon; Spinach Salad with Pan-Roasted Lamb Chops; Bok Choy Salad with Pan-Seared Tofu; Pan-Roasted Rib Eyes; and Pan-Roasted Chicken Breasts.

Recharge Recipes

(8-Hour Window)

Colla-Holla Latte

What do you get when you combine a hint of hot chocolate, almond, and coconut flavors with coffee and collagen? The best drink ever! Terry MUST have coffee in the morning, and this and the Morning Glory Coffee (page 111) are both his faves, which he interchanges depending on his mood.

SERVES 1

8 ounces freshly brewed coffee

1 tablespoon coconut oil

1 tablespoon cacao butter

1 tablespoon almond butter

2 drops stevia

1 scoop Colla-Holla or
1 tablespoon grass-fed collagen

1. Add coffee, coconut oil, butters, and stevia to a blender, and blend for 1 minute at high speed.

2. Add Colla-Holla and blend for another 10 seconds.

3. Transfer to your favorite coffee cup and enjoy!

Morning Glory Coffee

Kick up the fat and protein in your favorite morning beverage with this blended brew. Enjoy warm for maximum taste.

SERVES 1

2 ounces freshly brewed espresso

6 ounces hot water

1 tablespoon grass-fed unsalted butter

1 tablespoon MCT oil

1 scoop protein powder, whey or plant

1 tablespoon raw cacao

1. Add all ingredients to a blender, and blend at high speed until all ingredients are completely emulsified.

2. Transfer to your favorite coffee mug and enjoy!

Iced Coffee

Ghee is a type of clarified butter that adds a tasty richness to this iced coffee treat. Don't skip the cinnamon! Heather loves this iced coffee for a midday break, but she prefers it with decaf.

SERVES 1

8 ounces freshly brewed coffee

1 tablespoon grass-fed ghee

1 tablespoon MCT oil

1/4 teaspoon Himalayan pink salt

1/2 teaspoon Ceylon cinnamon

1. Add all ingredients to a blender, and blend at high speed until all ingredients are completely emulsified.

2. Pour over ice in a glass and enjoy!

Blended Iced Coffee with Coconut Whipped Cream

If you're craving a sweet coffee treat, this is the one you want! Heather loves this yummy blended drink as a dessert (always with decaf for her!).

SERVES 1

Coconut Whipped Cream

1 can coconut milk, full fat   2 drops stevia

Blended Iced Coffee

12 ounces freshly brewed coffee   4 drops stevia

1 tablespoon grass-fed ghee   1/4 teaspoon vanilla extract

1 tablespoon MCT oil   1/4 teaspoon Ceylon cinnamon

1 tablespoon raw almond butter   6 ice cubes

1 tablespoon cacao butter

1. Chill the can of coconut milk in the refrigerator overnight. Once chilled, drain the liquid from the can and add the fat and the stevia to a small bowl or the bowl of your stand mixer. Whip at high speed until peaks form, 2 to 3 minutes. Transfer the whipped cream to a glass container and refrigerate until ready to use.

2. Add the blended iced coffee ingredients to a blender, and blend at high speed until all ingredients are well blended.

3. Pour the coffee into a serving glass, top it with 2 tablespoons of coconut whipped cream, and enjoy!

Roasted Cauliflower Hummus

This remixed version of hummus is low-carb friendly and packed with flavor. Enjoy it with our Crispy Okra Chips (page 115) or Golden Baked Zucchini Chips (page 116), just like Terry would as a fun snack to share with the kids!

SERVES 8

1 large head cauliflower

3 tablespoons olive oil

¼ cup tahini

2 tablespoons fresh lemon juice

½ tablespoon chopped shallots

1 teaspoon sea salt

½ teaspoon ground cumin

¼ teaspoon ground black pepper

2 tablespoons chopped Kalamata olives

2 tablespoons crumbled feta cheese

1 tablespoon finely chopped fresh cilantro

1. Preheat the oven to 400°F.

2. Trim the cauliflower, and cut into small florets, removing the core. Toss with 1 tablespoon of the olive oil and spread evenly across a baking sheet.

3. Roast the cauliflower until fork tender, about 30 minutes, rotating the pan front to back halfway through cooking.

4. When cool enough to handle, transfer the cauliflower to a food processor. Add the tahini, lemon juice, shallots, sea salt, cumin, pepper, and remaining 2 tablespoons olive oil. Blend all the ingredients until smooth, adding 1 to 2 tablespoons of water to adjust the hummus to your desired consistency.

5. Serve garnished with chopped olives, feta, and cilantro.

Crispy Okra Chips

Though okra is known to be more of a soft-textured Southern staple, these okra chips are light, airy, and crisp. To ensure their texture, be sure to rinse the okra thoroughly after the vinegar wash and do not overcrowd the pan when baking. Serve the okra chips with Roasted Cauliflower Hummus (page 114) or enjoy as a stand-alone snack!

SERVES 4

1 pound okra, rinsed

1 tablespoon distilled white vinegar

1 tablespoon olive oil

1 teaspoon La Baleine Kosher Sea Salt

$\frac{1}{2}$ teaspoon garlic powder

$\frac{1}{2}$ teaspoon paprika

$\frac{1}{2}$ teaspoon ground white pepper

1. Preheat the oven to 500°F. Line a baking sheet with foil.

2. Slice the okra pods lengthwise. Place the sliced okra pods in a large bowl and add water to cover completely. Add the vinegar and mix well. Let the okra stand for 20 minutes, stirring every 5 minutes. Drain and rinse the okra pods under cold water and pat dry with a clean kitchen towel.

3. In a large bowl, toss the okra with the olive oil, kosher salt, garlic powder, paprika, and white pepper until evenly coated.

4. Arrange the okra on the foil-lined sheet and bake for 15 minutes, flipping over halfway through the cooking time.

5. Remove the okra from the oven and reduce the oven temperature to 170°F. When the oven has cooled, return the baking sheet to the oven and prop the oven door ajar. Bake the okra until crisp, 2 to 2½ hours. Remove the okra from the oven and cool for 30 minutes.

Golden Baked Zucchini Chips

These chips are a great crowd-pleaser! Use the spice blend we've included here or create your own flavors. The possibilities are endless! Serve the zucchini chips alone or enjoy as a side with a Bacon-Wrapped Breakfast Burger (page 127).

SERVES 4

2 large zucchini, rinsed and dried

La Baleine Kosher Sea Salt

Chip Spice

1 teaspoon La Baleine Kosher Sea Salt

$\frac{1}{2}$ teaspoon ground white pepper

$\frac{1}{2}$ teaspoon garlic powder

Cooking spray

$\frac{1}{2}$ teaspoon paprika

1 tablespoon olive oil

1. Using a mandoline, slice the zucchini into $\frac{1}{8}$-inch-thick rounds and arrange the rounds in a single layer on a clean kitchen towel. Sprinkle the rounds with kosher salt and cover with another clean kitchen towel. Place a baking sheet on top of the zucchini rounds and weight it down with a cutting board or plate to press out any excess water. Allow to stand for 20 to 25 minutes, applying pressure every so often.

2. Meanwhile, make the chip spice: In a small bowl, mix together the kosher salt, garlic powder, paprika, and white pepper and set aside.

3. Preheat the oven to 225°F. Line several baking sheets with parchment paper. Lightly coat the parchment paper with cooking spray.

4. Arrange the zucchini rounds in a single layer on the baking sheets, fitting as many as possible. Lightly brush the tops of the zucchini with the olive oil. Sprinkle the chip spice over the zucchini rounds.

5. Bake the zucchini rounds until crispy and golden brown, 1½ to 2 hours, rotating the pan front to back 45 minutes into cooking. Transfer the zucchini chips to paper towels to cool and to absorb excess oil. If some chips are uncooked, just place them back in the oven for a little longer.

Killer Kale Chips

One of Max's (the Dubrows' oldest daughter) favorite things is this recipe! We love to multiply this recipe and prep enough chips for the week. Store them in airtight containers or pre-portion them in zip-seal bags for a quick snack on the go! Enjoy with our Avocado Hummus (page 159).

SERVES 4

1 pound kale, cleaned and chopped

2 tablespoons ghee

2 teaspoons lemon juice

1 teaspoon garlic powder

½ teaspoon ground black pepper

1 teaspoon La Baleine Kosher Sea Salt

1 ounce parmesan cheese, finely grated

1. Preheat the oven to 275°.

2. Toss the kale into a large bowl, and massage it with ghee and lemon juice for 5 to 7 minutes.

3. Season the kale with garlic powder, pepper, salt, and parmesan cheese.

4. Spread the kale in an even layer on a baking sheet, and place it in the oven.

5. Bake until slightly crisp, 20 to 25 minutes, and be sure to rotate the pan halfway through your cooking time.

6. Allow to cool for 3 to 5 minutes.

Deviled Eggs, 3 Ways

One of Heather's favorite snacks, these deviled eggs are an excellent accompaniment to your favorite glass of bubbly! For a super-luxe cheat day, top your smoked salmon and dill deviled eggs with caviar.

SERVES 4

6 large cage-free eggs

1 teaspoon baking soda

Ice water

Plain

½ cup plain whole-milk Greek yogurt

1 tablespoon Dijon mustard

1 teaspoon sea salt

½ teaspoon ground white pepper

Smoked paprika, for garnish

Bacon & Parmesan

2 slices uncured bacon, cooked and chopped or crumbled

1 ounce parmesan cheese, shredded

Smoked Salmon & Dill

2 ounces smoked salmon, chopped

½ tablespoon finely chopped fresh dill

1. In a saucepan, combine the eggs, water to cover by 1 inch, and the baking soda. Bring to a boil and then boil for 1 minute. Cover, remove from the heat, and let sit covered for 12 minutes. Meanwhile, fill a medium bowl with ice water.

2. Drain the eggs and submerge them in the ice water to cool completely. (If not using right away, store the eggs in the refrigerator.) Carefully crack the eggs and remove the shells. Slice them in half lengthwise and remove the yolks to a separate bowl.

3. **For the plain deviled eggs:** Mash the egg yolks with the yogurt, mustard, salt, and white pepper. Pipe or scoop the yolk mixture back into the egg whites and sprinkle with smoked paprika to garnish.

For the bacon & parmesan eggs: Prepare the plain deviled egg filling and mash in the bacon and parmesan, reserving some for garnish. Fill the egg whites as directed above and garnish with the reserved bacon, parmesan, and smoked paprika.

For the smoked salmon & dill eggs: Prepare the plain deviled egg filling and mash in the smoked salmon and dill, reserving some for garnish. Fill the egg whites as directed above and garnish with the reserved smoked salmon, dill, and smoked paprika.

Loaded Celery Sticks

This cool, crunchy snack is a family favorite and sure to please any crowd you're entertaining. Whether you're serving these for game day or an afternoon snack, you can prep the filling a few days in advance for an easy-to-build appetizer!

SERVES 8 TO 10

1 bunch celery, rinsed and drained, ends trimmed

1 cup plain whole-milk Greek yogurt

2 tablespoons MCT oil

3/4 cup chopped dill pickles

6 slices uncured bacon, cooked and chopped or crumbled

1/2 tablespoon chopped fresh parsley

1 teaspoon sea salt

1/2 teaspoon garlic powder

1/2 teaspoon onion powder

1/4 teaspoon dried dill

1/4 teaspoon chopped fresh dill

1. Halve the celery stalks so that they are about 4 inches in length.

2. In a medium bowl, stir together the yogurt, MCT oil, pickles, bacon, parsley, sea salt, garlic powder, and onion powder.

3. Using a spoon, fill each celery stalk with the filling and garnish with the dill.

Fat Bomb Burger Sliders with Bacon-Wrapped Onion Rings

The whole family loves this one! You can't lose with these juicy burgers paired with bacon-wrapped onion rings. Level up the keto-friendly flavor with our sugar-free ketchup (page 148).

SERVES 5 OR 6

Cooking spray

Bacon-Wrapped Onion Rings

3 yellow onions

24 slices uncured bacon

Sliders

1 pound grass-fed ground beef

1 tablespoon La Baleine Kosher Sea Salt

$1/2$ teaspoon garlic powder

$1/2$ teaspoon onion powder

$1/2$ teaspoon paprika

$1/2$ teaspoon dried thyme

$1/2$ teaspoon ground black pepper

$1/2$ cup chopped fresh basil

2 tablespoons grass-fed unsalted butter, melted

$1/4$ cup shredded mozzarella cheese

2 Roma (plum) tomatoes, sliced, for serving

10 butter lettuce leaves, for serving

1. Preheat the oven to 375°F. Line a rimmed baking sheet with foil and coat lightly with cooking spray. Coat 8 to 10 cups (depending on the size of the cups in your pan) of a mini muffin pan with cooking spray.

2. Make the onion rings: Slice the onions into ½-inch-thick rings, separate 24 larger rings (no smaller circumference than the bacon in hand), and reserve the rest for stock, other recipes, or freeze for future use.

3. Wrap each onion ring with bacon securely but not too tightly, leaving room for the bacon to cook down in size. Fold the ends of the bacon pieces on the bottom or inside of the onion and secure the ends with water-soaked toothpicks.

4. Arrange the wrapped onion rings on the prepared baking sheet and bake until golden and crispy, about 30 minutes, rotating the pan front to back halfway through cooking. When done, drain on paper towels.

5. Meanwhile, make the sliders: In a medium bowl, combine the ground beef, salt, garlic powder, onion powder, paprika, thyme, pepper, basil, and melted butter. Fold in the mozzarella.

6. Press 2 to 3 tablespoons seasoned beef into each muffin cup. Bake until the meat has reached desired doneness, about 15 minutes for well-done.

7. Serve the sliders with the tomato slices, butter lettuce, and onion rings!

Breakfast Salad with Ranch Dressing

Even if you're not a "breakfast person," you've got to have some mid-morning fuel to break your fast! Take a tip from Terry and Max by turning the foods you love into breakfast.

SERVES 2

Ranch Dressing

$1/2$ cup avocado oil mayonnaise

$1/2$ cup plain whole-milk Greek yogurt

$1/4$ cup heavy (whipping) cream

2 tablespoons distilled white vinegar

1 tablespoon chopped fresh parsley

1 teaspoon chopped fresh chives

3 tablespoons fresh dill, or 1 tablespoon dried

1 teaspoon onion powder

1 teaspoon garlic powder

1 teaspoon La Baleine Kosher Sea Salt

$1/2$ teaspoon ground black pepper

Breakfast Salad

2 romaine lettuce hearts

2 tablespoons chopped walnuts

$1/2$ medium avocado, scooped into chunks

2 ounces radish sprouts

1 ounce feta cheese, crumbled

1 tablespoon olive oil

2 large cage-free eggs

Salt and ground black pepper

1. Make the ranch dressing: In a medium bowl, vigorously whisk together the mayo, yogurt, cream, vinegar, herbs, onion powder, garlic powder, salt, and pepper. Refrigerate until ready to serve.

2. Make the breakfast salad: Wash and rinse the lettuce thoroughly with cold water, then chop and dry in a salad spinner. Divide the lettuce between individual serving plates or bowls. Dividing evenly, top the salads with the walnuts, avocado chunks, radish sprouts, and feta crumbles.

3. In a nonstick skillet, heat the olive oil over medium-low heat until the oil is slightly shimmering, 2 to 3 minutes. Crack the eggs into a small ramekin one at a time and carefully add them on opposite sides of the skillet. Reduce the heat to low and cover with a tight lid. Cook the eggs undisturbed until the whites are set but the yolks are still runny, about 2 minutes.

4. Carefully, use a spatula to top each salad with an egg and season with salt and pepper to taste. Drizzle the salads with 2 to 3 tablespoons of ranch dressing and serve immediately. Store the remaining dressing in an airtight glass container in the refrigerator for up to 7 days.

Cast-Iron Skillet Frittata

Shut your next brunch down with this killer dish as a main or side. This frittata is easy to build and rich in fat and flavor. The bonus is that you can serve it straight from the skillet!

SERVES 4

12 large cage-free eggs

1/4 cup heavy (whipping) cream

1 tablespoon MCT oil

1 teaspoon sea salt

1/2 teaspoon ground white pepper

8 slices uncured bacon, diced

1 tablespoon ghee

2 cups sliced shiitake mushroom caps

1/2 cup arugula

1 cup shaved parmesan cheese

1. Preheat the oven to 355°F.

2. In a medium bowl, whisk together the eggs, cream, MCT oil, sea salt, and white pepper. Set aside.

3. Place a large cast-iron skillet over medium heat. Add the bacon and sauté for 3 to 4 minutes. Add the ghee and mushrooms and, stirring frequently, sauté the bacon and mushrooms in butter for another 3 minutes, until the mushrooms have browned. (Keep medium heat levels by adjusting your heat as needed.)

4. Add the arugula and cook until just wilted, 1 to 2 minutes. Remove the skillet from the heat and sprinkle the parmesan evenly over the sautéed ingredients. Pour the egg mixture over the ingredients in the skillet.

5. Transfer the skillet to the oven and bake until the egg no longer jiggles, 20 to 25 minutes.

6. Let the frittata cool for 5 to 7 minutes before slicing.

Parmesan & Dill Blinis
with Smoked Salmon

One of Heather's favorite finger foods to pair with a crisp, cool glass of champs! These are also lovely paired with a French burgundy white wine.

SERVES 4

3 large cage-free eggs, at room temperature

$1/4$ cup heavy (whipping) cream

$1/2$ teaspoon white balsamic vinegar

$1^1/2$ cups almond flour

$1/2$ teaspoon baking soda

1 teaspoon sea salt

$1/4$ teaspoon ground white pepper

$1/2$ cup shaved parmesan cheese

1 tablespoon chopped fresh dill

1 tablespoon ghee

12 ounces smoked salmon, sliced

1. Preheat a griddle over medium heat.

2. In a blender or food processor, blend together the eggs, cream, and vinegar. Add the almond flour, baking soda, salt, white pepper, and $1/4$ cup of the parmesan. Cover and process for 1 minute. Fold in the remaining parmesan and $1/2$ tablespoon of the dill.

3. Grease the heated griddle with the ghee.

4. Ladle the batter onto the griddle in about 2-inch rounds. When a blini begins to bubble, flip and cook the second side. Repeat until all the batter is used.

5. To serve, top evenly with smoked salmon and garnish with the remaining chopped dill.

Bacon-Wrapped Breakfast Burgers

These brunch-style burgers are a mimosa's best friend! Even if you don't eat these protein- and fat-packed burgers for breakfast, they make a great lunch or dinner paired with our Golden Baked Zucchini Chips (page 116).

SERVES 6

1 medium zucchini

La Baleine Kosher Sea Salt

12 slices uncured bacon

Cooking spray

1½ pounds grass-fed ground beef

3 garlic cloves, minced

2 tablespoons finely chopped fresh parsley

2 tablespoons finely chopped fresh chives

2 tablespoons ghee, melted

Ground black pepper

6 tablespoons olive oil

6 large cage-free eggs

Ketchup (page 148), for serving

1. Using the largest holes on a box grater, shred the zucchini. Place the shredded zucchini in a clean kitchen towel and squeeze to remove moisture. Lightly salt the zucchini and set aside wrapped in the kitchen towel.

2. Meanwhile, arrange the bacon on a microwave-safe plate lined with paper towels and cover with another paper towel. Microwave on high until cooked but not crispy, 2 to 3 minutes.

3. Line a baking sheet with foil and coat with cooking spray. Lay pairs of bacon strips in an X on the baking sheet. You should have 6 of them. Set aside.

4. Position a rack 4 inches from the heating element and preheat the broiler.

5. Wring out the zucchini one last time and transfer to a large bowl. Add the beef, garlic, parsley, chives, ghee, ½ tablespoon salt, and 1 teaspoon pepper. Mix well, then shape into 6 patties, making sure

to press into the centers of the patties to keep the shaping. Place a patty on the center of each bacon X and wrap the strips around patties. Secure the bacon strips with water-soaked toothpicks.

6. Broil the bacon burgers for about 6 minutes for rare to medium rare, or longer depending on your desired level of doneness. Let the burgers rest while you prepare the eggs. Remove the toothpicks.

7. In a nonstick skillet, heat 2 tablespoons of the olive oil over medium-low heat until the oil is slightly shimmering, 2 to 3 minutes. Cooking 2 eggs at a time, crack the eggs into a small ramekin one at a time and carefully add them on opposite sides of the skillet. Reduce the heat to low and cover with a tight lid. Cook the eggs undisturbed until the whites are set but the yolks are still runny, about 2 minutes. Repeat with the remaining oil and eggs.

8. Carefully, use a spatula to top each burger with an egg and season with salt and pepper to taste. Serve with our Dubrow-friendly ketchup and enjoy!

Cauliflower Bacon Hash
with Soft-Boiled Eggs

This is one of my favorite dishes to make for the family when we have "breakfast for dinner." The yolk from the soft-boiled eggs is the perfect sauce! This dish is a great main for adults and as a topping for the kids' avocado toasts. You can also enjoy the hash and eggs topped with our Hollandaise (page 192).

SERVES 4

8 slices uncured bacon. chopped

2 tablespoons ghee

1 pound cauliflower, cut into small pieces

1 garlic clove, minced

2 fresh red jalapeños, seeded and minced

1 teaspoon sea salt

$1/2$ teaspoon ground white pepper

$1/2$ teaspoon paprika

$1/2$ teaspoon onion powder

$1/4$ cup Keto Bone Broth (page 147)

Chopped fresh parsley, for garnish

4 soft-boiled eggs (see directions on page 130)

1. In a skillet, cook the bacon over medium-low heat until the fat is rendered and the bacon is crispy, 10 to 12 minutes. Remove the bacon from the skillet and leave the rendered fat in the pan.

2. Add the ghee to the pan and melt over medium-high heat. Add the cauliflower and cook until golden brown, 2 to 3 minutes. Add the garlic, jalapeños, salt, white pepper, paprika, and onion powder. Add the keto broth, cover, and cook until the cauliflower is fork tender, 2 to 3 more minutes. Remove the cover in the last minute of cooking to reduce the liquid.

3. Return the bacon to the skillet and toss well. Remove from the heat. Serve topped with fresh parsley and soft-boiled eggs.

Soft-Boiled Eggs: Fill a medium saucepan halfway with water and heat to a rolling boil. With a slotted spoon, gently lower the eggs into the boiling water one at a time. Set a timer for 6 minutes. Once the timer is up, carefully drain the hot water and run cold water over the eggs to halt the cooking process. Carefully peel the eggs and serve while still hot.

Arugula Salad with Crispy Pan-Roasted Salmon

This fast and tasty dish is perfect for busy weeknights and work lunches. Batch-prepare a few of our salad dressings and double this recipe for four ready-to-go lunches.

SERVES 2

Pan-Roasted Salmon

1 tablespoon grapeseed oil

2 skin-on wild-caught salmon fillets (4 ounces each)

1 teaspoon sea salt

1/2 teaspoon ground black pepper

2 tablespoons grass-fed unsalted butter

4 sprigs fresh thyme

1 garlic clove, smashed

Arugula Salad

2 cups arugula, rinsed and dried

1/2 medium avocado, scooped into chunks

2 tablespoons chopped walnuts

2 to 3 tablespoons salad dressing: Red Wine Vinaigrette (page 149), White Wine Vinaigrette (page 150), or Asian-Style Vinaigrette (page 151)

1. Chill two serving bowls in the freezer. Preheat the oven to 400°F.

2. Make the salmon: In a large ovenproof skillet, heat the grapeseed oil over medium-high heat. Season the salmon fillets with the salt and pepper. Add to the skillet skin-side down and cook undisturbed until the skin crisps and the bottom of the fish starts to turn opaque, 3 to 4 minutes. Add the butter, thyme, and garlic to the pan and cook, basting the fillets, for 1 minute.

3. Transfer the pan to the oven and cook for 3 minutes for medium-well, or more depending on your desired level of doneness. Be sure to baste once before removing the fish from the oven.

4. Meanwhile, make the salad: In a bowl, toss together the arugula, avocado chunks, and walnuts. Divide between the chilled serving bowls.

5. Serve the salmon skin-side up over the salads and drizzle with your choice of approved dressings.

Spinach Salad with Pan-Roasted Lamb Chops

A little bit of Heather and a little bit of Terry make this salad a match made in heaven. Terry loves a fresh spinach salad while Heather is always in the mood for an on-the-rare-side lamb chop. Enjoy this one with our Red Wine Vinaigrette (page 149).

SERVES 2

Pan-Roasted Lamb Chops

4 lamb loin chops

2 tablespoons grapeseed oil

1 teaspoon sea salt

$1/2$ teaspoon ground black pepper

2 tablespoons grass-fed unsalted butter

4 sprigs fresh thyme

1 garlic clove, smashed

Spinach Salad

2 cups spinach

$1/4$ cup sliced cherry tomatoes

8 Kalamata olives, chopped

$1/2$ green bell pepper, sliced

$1/4$ cup shaved parmesan cheese

2 to 3 tablespoons salad dressing: Red Wine Vinaigrette (page 149), White Wine Vinaigrette (page 150), or Asian-Style Vinaigrette (page 151)

1. Chill two serving bowls in the freezer.

2. Cook the lamb chops: Remove the lamb chops from the fridge 20 to 30 minutes before cooking,

3. In a large skillet, heat the grapeseed oil over medium-high heat. Season the lamb chops with the salt and pepper. Cook the chops undisturbed for 3 to 4 minutes on each side, or until they are caramelized and browned on each side.

4. Add the butter, thyme, and garlic to the pan and cook, basting the lamb chops, for 1 to 2 minutes for medium-rare. (If a further doneness is desired, cook for 3 to 4 minutes longer for medium-well.) Remove the lamb chops from the heat and place on a plate to rest.

5. Meanwhile, make the salad: In a bowl, toss together the spinach, tomatoes, olives, bell peppers, and parmesan. Divide between the chilled serving bowls.

6. Serve the rested lamb chops over the salads and drizzle with your choice of approved salad dressing.

Grilled Spatchcock Chicken & Cauliflower Stuffing

Winner, winner, chicken dinner! Literally, this dinner is always a winner at Château Dubrow, as the kids and parents alike love this recipe. Add a layer of flavor to your version by incorporating alder or applewood smoking chips to your grill.

SERVES 6 TO 8

1 whole roasting chicken (4 to 7 pounds)

$1/4$ cup olive oil

Grated zest and juice of 1 lemon

$1/2$ tablespoon chopped fresh rosemary

$3/4$ teaspoon chopped fresh thyme

2 teaspoons ground black pepper

2 teaspoons paprika

1 teaspoon garlic powder

1 teaspoon onion powder

$1^1/2$ tablespoons La Baleine Kosher Sea Salt

Cauliflower Stuffing

4 tablespoons grass-fed unsalted butter

4 celery stalks, diced

1 medium onion, diced

1 head cauliflower, cut into $1/2$-inch florets

$1/2$ cup chopped portobello mushrooms

1 teaspoon sea salt

1 teaspoon ground black pepper

2 tablespoons finely chopped fresh parsley

$1/2$ tablespoon finely chopped fresh rosemary

$1/2$ cup Keto Bone Broth (page 147)

1. Preheat a grill to medium-high.

2. Place the chicken breast-side down on a cutting board with the neck end facing toward you. Remove the backbone with kitchen shears by cutting along both sides from end to end. Flip the chicken and open it like a book. Use a chef's knife to score down the sternum. This will make it easier to pop out the breast bone and flatten the chicken. Use your palms to press firmly on the breasts. The chicken should be evenly flat on both sides.

3. In a small bowl, mix together the olive oil, lemon zest, lemon juice, herbs, pepper, paprika, garlic powder, and onion powder. Brush the chicken all over with the seasoned olive oil.

4. Just before grilling, salt the chicken all over. Place the chicken on the grill, breast-side down, over direct heat and close the grill. Grill for 12 to 15 minutes, rotating the chicken halfway through cooking. Turn the chicken over and grill for another 12 to 15 minutes, rotating the chicken halfway through. Reduce the heat to maintain a temperature of 350°F and grill over indirect heat until the internal temperature reaches 165°F, another 12 to 15 minutes.

5. Meanwhile, make the cauliflower stuffing: In a large skillet, melt the butter over medium heat. Add the celery and onion to the skillet and cook until the onions are translucent, 4 to 5 minutes. Add the cauliflower and mushrooms, season with the salt and pepper, and cook until fork tender, 7 to 8 minutes. Add the parsley, rosemary, and bone broth. Cook uncovered until all of the vegetables are tender, and the liquid is absorbed, 3 to 4 minutes.

6. Remove the chicken from the grill and allow it to rest. Slice and serve the chicken with the cauliflower stuffing. Save the juices from the cutting board for additional flavor!

Southern-Style Shrimp & Cauliflower "Grits"

Fun fact: Some of Terry's favorite dishes that I make are the ones most heavily influenced by the South. This lightened version of a Southern classic is great for a cozy evening or potluck among friends!

SERVES 4

$\frac{1}{2}$ teaspoon sea salt

$\frac{1}{4}$ teaspoon garlic powder

$\frac{1}{4}$ teaspoon paprika

$\frac{1}{4}$ teaspoon ground black pepper

$\frac{1}{4}$ teaspoon cayenne pepper

$\frac{1}{4}$ teaspoon dried oregano

$\frac{1}{4}$ teaspoon dried thyme

$\frac{1}{4}$ teaspoon onion powder

$\frac{1}{4}$ teaspoon red pepper flakes

1 pound wild-caught shrimp, peeled and deveined

$\frac{1}{2}$ tablespoon ghee, melted

1 head cauliflower

2 tablespoons grass-fed unsalted butter

1 tablespoon minced shallots

$1\frac{1}{2}$ cups Keto Bone Broth (page 147)

$\frac{1}{2}$ cup plain whole-milk Greek yogurt

$\frac{1}{2}$ cup grated parmesan cheese

4 ounces pancetta

1 tablespoon olive oil

2 links andouille chicken sausage, diced

$\frac{1}{2}$ tablespoon arrowroot powder

3 tablespoons finely chopped fresh parsley

1. In a large bowl, mix together the salt, garlic powder, paprika, black pepper, cayenne, oregano, thyme, onion powder, and pepper flakes. Add the shrimp and ghee, and toss, making sure to coat all the shrimp well.

2. Process the cauliflower into "rice" with a grater, food processor, or spiralizer.

3. In a shallow saucepan, melt the butter over medium-high heat. Add the shallots and sauté for 45 seconds to 1 minute, or until just translucent. Stir in $\frac{3}{4}$ cup of the broth and bring to a boil. Whisk in the yogurt and then add the parmesan little bit by little bit. Continue stirring until the ingredients are well incorporated. Add

the riced cauliflower and cook for 2 more minutes. Reduce the heat and keep warm.

4. Set a cast-iron or nonstick skillet over medium-low heat. Add the pancetta and cook to slowly render the fat. When the pancetta is crispy, remove the crisped pieces and leave the fat in the pan.

5. Add the olive oil to the pancetta fat over medium-high heat. Add the seasoned shrimp and sear on both sides until the shrimp are bright pink and opaque. Set the shrimp aside on a plate.

6. Add the chicken sausage and cook until the sausage is browned, 2 to 3 minutes. Add the arrowroot powder and whisk in the remaining ¾ cup bone broth. Bring to a boil to thicken the sauce. Return the pancetta and shrimp to the pan. Stir in the parsley.

7. Serve the shrimp and sausage on top of the cauliflower "grits," with spoonfuls of the pan gravy. Enjoy!

Crispy Chicken Wings with Spicy Mustard Greens

The secret to making the flavor pop on these wings is to not skip the pickle juice marinade. If you want to bring your A game to the next Super Bowl party, these should absolutely be the dish you make!

You can also prepare these with chicken tenderloins rather than party wings. Just knock your cooking time down to 10 to 12 minutes on each side.

SERVES 4

1 pound chicken wings, separated and tips removed

2 cups pickle juice

$^1/_2$ tablespoon La Baleine Kosher Sea Salt

1 teaspoon ground black pepper

1 teaspoon garlic powder

1 teaspoon onion powder

$^1/_2$ teaspoon chili powder

$^1/_2$ teaspoon paprika

Cooking spray

2 tablespoons grapeseed oil

Spicy Mustard Greens

3 bunches mustard greens

1 tablespoon olive oil

1 teaspoon sea salt

2 tablespoons coconut oil

1 tablespoon mustard seeds

$^1/_2$ shallot, sliced

2 serrano chiles, sliced

1 tablespoon minced fresh ginger

10 Thai basil leaves, chopped

1 teaspoon grated lime zest

Ranch Dressing (page 123), for serving

1. Place the chicken wings in a large zip-seal bag and cover with the pickle juice. Massage the bag to coat the chicken well and let the wings marinate for 3 hours in the refrigerator.

2. In a small bowl, combine the salt, pepper, garlic powder, onion powder, chili powder, and paprika and set aside.

3. Once the wings are finished marinating, preheat the oven to 400°F. Line a large rimmed baking sheet with foil. Set a wire rack in the pan and coat with cooking spray.

4. Drain the wings in a colander and pat dry with paper towels. Toss the wings with the grapeseed oil and the reserved spice mix, making sure to coat all wings evenly.

5. Arrange the wings skin-side down on the rack in the pan and bake until they are golden brown and the skin is crisp, about 40 minutes, flipping the wings over halfway through.

6. Meanwhile, preheat a grill to high.

7. Prepare the mustard greens: Brush the mustard greens with the olive oil and season with the salt.

8. Grill the greens until they are blistered and charred, about 30 seconds on each side. Transfer to a baking sheet and remove any tough stems.

9. In a skillet, heat the coconut oil over medium-high heat. Add the mustards seeds and continuously move the skillet around until the seeds begin to pop, about 30 seconds. Increase the heat and add the shallots, chiles, ginger, basil, and lime zest. Cook until the shallots are golden, 2 to 3 minutes.

10. To serve, spoon the coconut mixture over the mustard greens and enjoy with crispy chicken wings and ranch dressing.

Bok Choy Salad with Pan-Seared Tofu

A great vegetarian option, this dish is also very quick and easy to make. Now that Max is a vegetarian, we're always looking for delicious options for her to pack for lunch on the go!

SERVES 2

Pan-Seared Tofu

1 block extra-firm tofu

2 tablespoons grapeseed oil

1 teaspoon sea salt

$1/2$ teaspoon ground black pepper

2 tablespoons grass-fed unsalted butter

4 sprigs fresh thyme

1 garlic clove, smashed

Bok Choy Salad

2 cups bok choy leaves

$1/4$ cup diced tomatoes

$1/4$ cup sliced fennel

1 celery stalk, diced

2 to 3 tablespoons salad dressing: Red Wine Vinaigrette (page 149), White Wine Vinaigrette (page 150), or Asian-Style Vinaigrette (page 151)

1. Chill two individual serving bowls in the freezer.

2. Prepare the tofu: Line a baking sheet with paper towels. Cut the tofu into 4 slices and place them on the paper towels. Place another set of paper towels over the tofu slices and top with another baking sheet. Use the top of the baking sheet to weight down the pan. "Press" the tofu for at least 30 minutes before cooking.

3. In a large skillet, heat the grapeseed oil over medium-high heat. Season the tofu with the salt and pepper. Add the tofu to the pan and cook undisturbed for 3 to 4 minutes on each side, or until tofu is caramelized and browned. Add the butter, thyme, and garlic to the pan and cook, basting the tofu, for 1 to 2 minutes.

4. Meanwhile, make the bok choy salad: In a bowl, combine the bok choy leaves, tomatoes, fennel, and celery. Toss well and divide between the chilled serving bowls.

5. Serve 2 tofu slices over each salad and drizzle with your choice of approved dressing.

Salmon & Avocado Poke
with Green "Noodle" Salad

Poke is so popular in Southern California that the recipes would have felt incomplete without a DKFD version! What's even better is that this recipe takes less than 30 minutes and requires no cooking.

SERVES 2

8 ounces skinless wild-caught salmon fillet, cut into small cubes

1 tablespoon sesame oil

2 teaspoons tamari

Green "Noodle" Salad

1 bunch collard greens, washed, and stems and midribs removed

1½ teaspoons sesame oil

¼ small head cabbage, core removed

For serving

½ medium avocado, sliced

1 teaspoon white sesame seeds

1 teaspoon black sesame seeds

2 teaspoons chopped fresh cilantro

½ medium zucchini, seeded and spiralized

½ green bell pepper, sliced

1 teaspoon sesame seeds

12 almonds, roughly chopped

Cilantro, for garnish

1. Chill two individual serving bowls in the freezer.

2. In a bowl, gently toss the salmon cubes with the sesame oil, tamari, both sesame seeds, and the cilantro. Cover with plastic wrap and set aside to marinate.

3. Stack the collard leaves, roll them up, and cut the bundles crosswise into thin slices. Transfer the collard strips to a bowl. Add the sesame oil and massage the collard strips until you feel them start to become more pliable, 5 to 7 minutes.

4. Shave or cut the cabbage into thin slices and add to the collard strips. Massage with the collards for 2 to 3 more minutes. Add the

zucchini noodles, bell pepper, sesame seeds, and almonds. Toss to evenly distribute all the ingredients.

5. To serve, divide the salad evenly between the chilled serving bowls. Top with the salmon poke and avocado slices and garnish with cilantro.

Roasted Garlic Butter Steak Bites with Italian Mustard Greens

SERVES 6

1 tablespoon olive oil

1½ pounds grass-fed sirloin steak, cubed

3 teaspoons sea salt

1 teaspoon coarsely ground black pepper

4 tablespoons grass-fed unsalted butter

5 cloves roasted garlic (page 146), minced

Italian Mustard Greens

2 tablespoons olive oil

2 cloves roasted garlic (page 146), minced

2 bunches mustard greens, stems removed and chopped

1 teaspoon coarsely ground black pepper

1 teaspoon crushed red pepper

1 tablespoon Red Wine Vinaigrette (page 149)

3 tablespoons Keto Bone Broth (page 147)

½ tablespoon stone-ground mustard

1. Heat the 1 tablespoon olive oil in a large skillet over medium-high heat. Sear the pieces of steak in a single layer until the outsides are browned or caramelized in color, 4 to 5 minutes. You may need to work in batches so as to not overcrowd the skillet. Sprinkle the steak with salt and pepper, and stir often. Remove the steak bites to a separate plate.

2. Reduce the heat to medium-low and melt the butter in the skillet. Stir the garlic into the pan, and cook for 1 minute, or until the garlic butter becomes very fragrant.

3. Add all the steak bites back to the pan. Stir to baste all the meat in garlic butter, and continue to cook for 1 to 2 more minutes. Reduce the heat to super low to keep the steak bites warm.

4. Meanwhile, make the Italian mustard greens: In another large skillet with sides, heat the 2 tablespoons olive oil over medium heat.

5. Add the garlic and sauté until very fragrant and tender, about 45 seconds to 1 minute.

6. Add the mustard greens to the skillet along with the peppers. Sauté until the greens begin to wilt, 1 to 2 minutes.

7. When the greens are wilted, add the vinaigrette and broth. Increase the heat to medium-high, and simmer until the greens are tender and the broth mostly reduced, 2 to 3 minutes.

8. Stir in the mustard and enjoy served underneath the steak bites and butter sauce!

ROASTED GARLIC

Makes 2 roasted garlic bulbs

2 whole garlic bulbs

2 tablespoons olive oil

2 teaspoons sea salt

1 teaspoon coarsely ground black pepper

1. Position an oven rack in the center of the oven and preheat the oven to 400°F.

2. Peel off the excess papery outside layers around the garlic bulbs, leaving the heads themselves intact.

3. With a sharp knife, cut ¼ inch off of the tops of the garlic bulbs, and place the garlic bulbs cut-side up on a sheet of aluminum foil.

4. Drizzle the garlic bulbs all over with olive oil, and season them with salt and pepper.

5. Wrap the garlic bulbs in foil, and bake them until very fragrant, 40 to 45 minutes. The garlic is done cooking when the middle is fork-tender. For deeper color and additional caramelization, cook the garlic longer, making sure to check it every 10 minutes to prevent burning.

6. Allow the garlic to cool slightly before handling. To remove the roasted cloves, press on the bottom of the bulbs to push them out of the paper. Serve or use immediately, or refrigerate them in an airtight container for up to 2 weeks.

Keto Bone Broth

Soup is life when fall hits at the Dubrow house, and I like to keep homemade stock on hand at all times. This bone broth is called for in numerous recipes, so don't be afraid of making too much! You can freeze this in ice cube trays for premeasured amounts of broth that you will then always have on hand for cooking.

SERVES 10

3 chicken carcasses (left over from roast chicken or from Grilled Spatchcock Chicken, page 135)

3 bay leaves

2 tablespoons black peppercorns

2 tablespoons apple cider vinegar

1 tablespoon ground turmeric

1 lemon, sliced

1. In a large stockpot, combine the chicken carcasses, bay leaves, peppercorns, and vinegar. Add 10 cups of water and bring to a boil. Reduce the heat to low, cover the pot, and simmer the stock for 24 to 48 hours. The stock is ready to use at 24 hours, but cooking for 48 hours will yield a richer stock.

2. Remove the broth from the heat and strain through a fine-mesh sieve into a pitcher or large bowl. Stir in the turmeric and lemon slices.

3. The broth can be consumed as a stand-alone beverage and also used for flavor in various recipes.

[]

Ketchup

We have to have ketchup, and this sugar-free version is the perfect accompaniment to our burgers!

MAKES ABOUT 4 CUPS

2 teaspoons olive oil

1 tablespoon minced shallots

1 (28-ounce) can tomato puree

¼ teaspoon cayenne pepper

1 tablespoon stevia

½ cup distilled white vinegar

1 cinnamon stick, broken

½ teaspoon whole cloves

½ teaspoon celery salt

La Baleine Kosher Sea Salt

1. In a medium saucepan, heat the olive oil over medium-low heat. Add the shallots and sauté until just translucent, 30 to 45 seconds. Add the tomato puree, cayenne, and stevia and simmer on low heat.

2. Meanwhile, in a small saucepan, combine the vinegar, cinnamon stick, whole cloves, and celery salt. Bring to a boil and remove from the heat. Strain the vinegar through a fine-mesh sieve (discard the solids).

3. Add the spiced vinegar to the tomato mixture. Simmer until ketchup consistency is achieved, 20 to 30 minutes. Salt to taste. Remove from the heat and allow to cool.

4. Transfer the ketchup to a food processor or blender and blend until smooth. Store in a glass container in the refrigerator for up to 3 weeks.

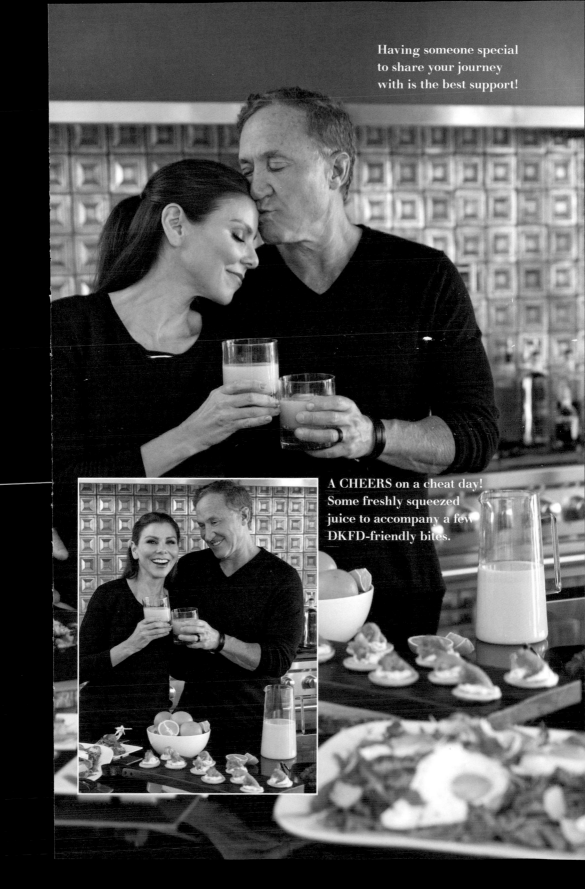

Having someone special to share your journey with is the best support!

A CHEERS on a cheat day! Some freshly squeezed juice to accompany a few DKFD-friendly bites.

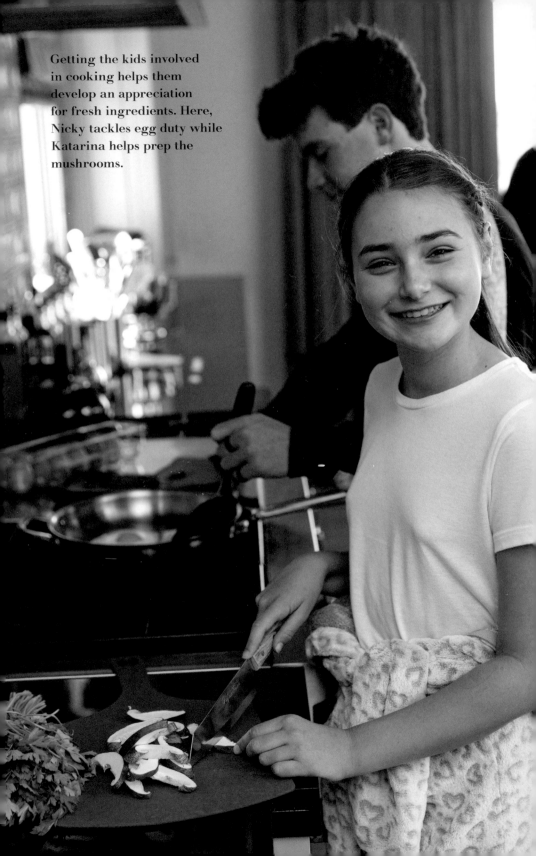

Getting the kids involved
in cooking helps them
develop an appreciation
for fresh ingredients. Here,
Nicky tackles egg duty while
Katarina helps prep the
mushrooms.

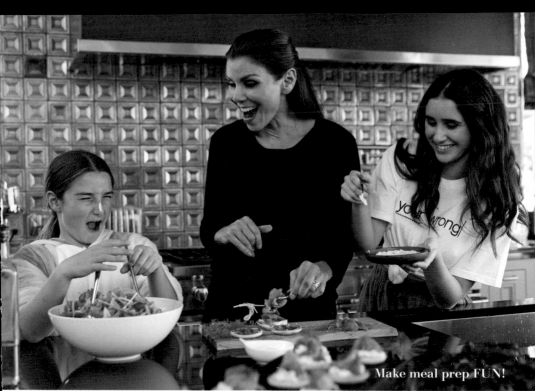

Make meal prep FUN!

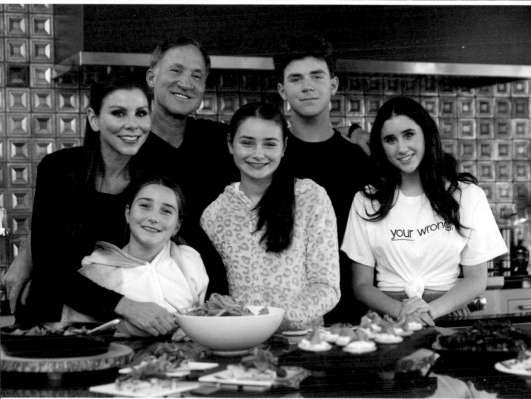

Family is everything.

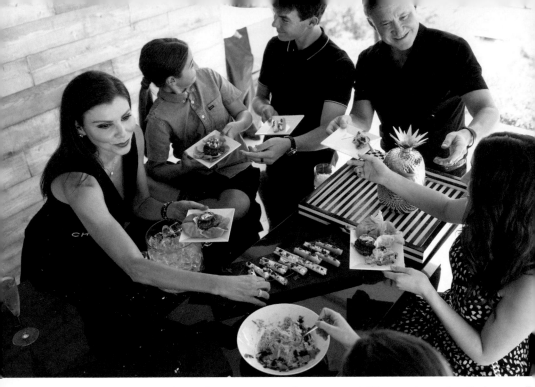

Where you eat can be as important as what you eat! Change it up by dining outside.

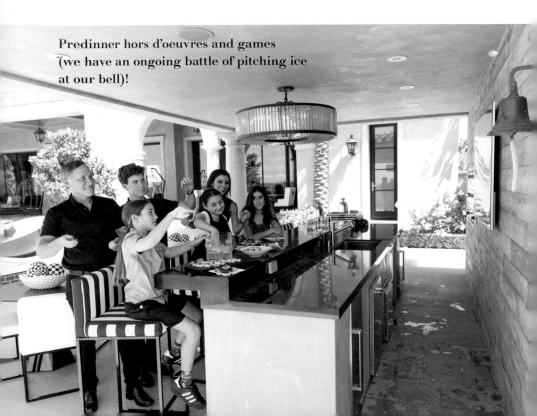

Predinner hors d'oeuvres and games (we have an ongoing battle of pitching ice at our bell)!

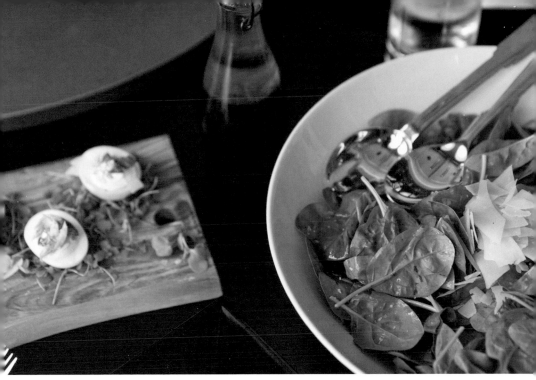

YUM! Our Bacon & Parmesan and Smoked Salmon & Dill Deviled Eggs (page 118) paired with a simple spinach and shaved parmesan salad (topped with our Red Wine Vinaigrette, page 149). Savory, satisfying food doesn't have to be complicated!

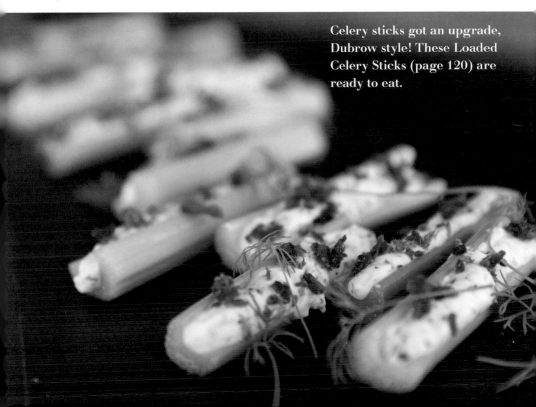

Celery sticks got an upgrade, Dubrow style! These Loaded Celery Sticks (page 120) are ready to eat.

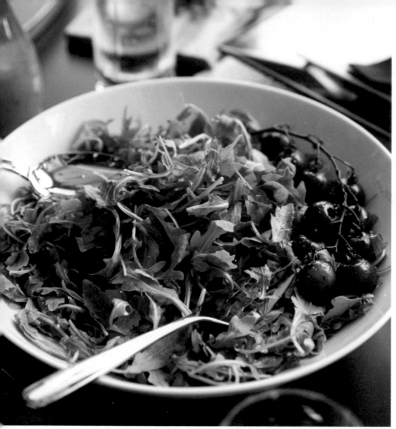

Make a batch of our White Wine Vinaigrette (page 150) ahead of time and use it to top any kind of fresh greens, such as one of our favorites: arugula.

Restaurant-quality Pan-Roasted Salmon (page 185) is a perfect dish for a busy night; it'll be on the table in less than 30 minutes!

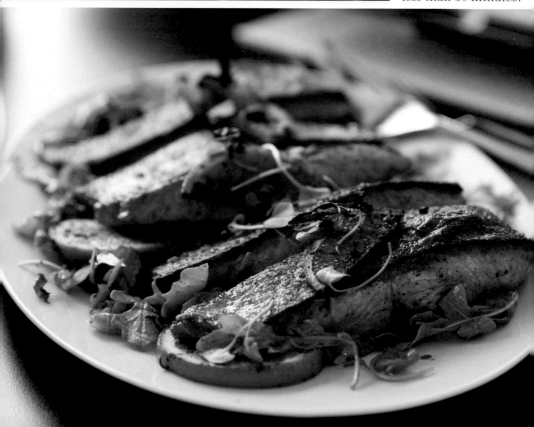

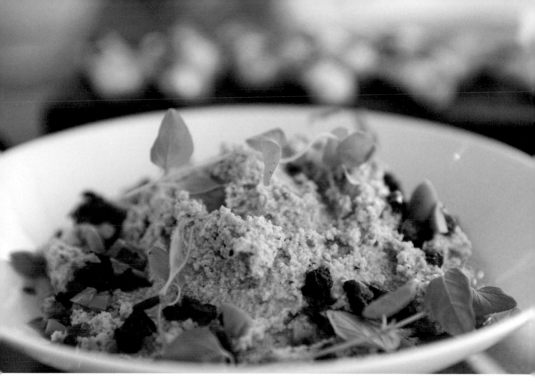

Most hummus is made from chickpeas, but we mix it up by using cauliflower (page 114)—be sure to give this one a try!

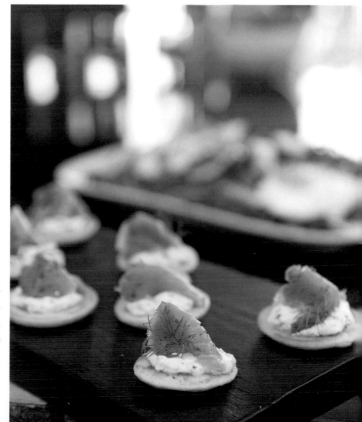

These Parmesan & Dill Blinis with Smoked Salmon (page 126) taste like a true treat!

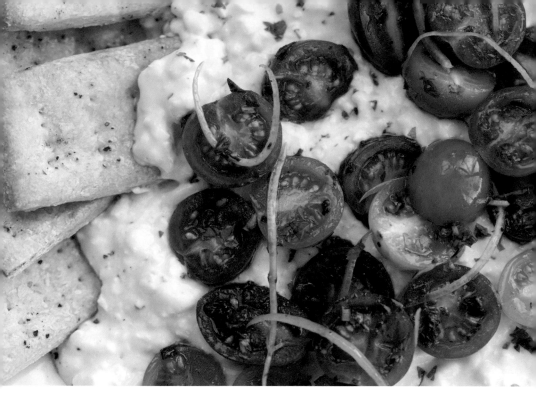

Let the DKFD introduce you to next-level snacking with bites like our Rosemary & Cracked Black Pepper Crackers (page 155) with Bruschetta Topping & Herbed Cottage Cheese (page 157).

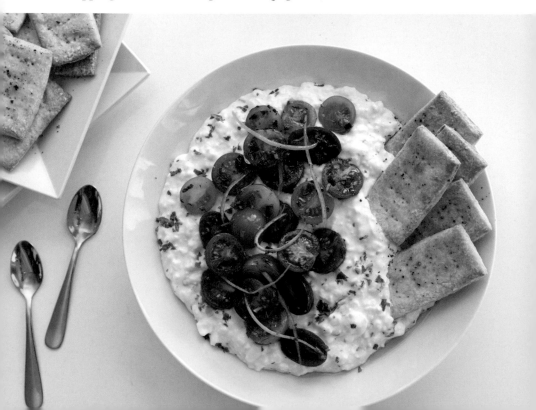

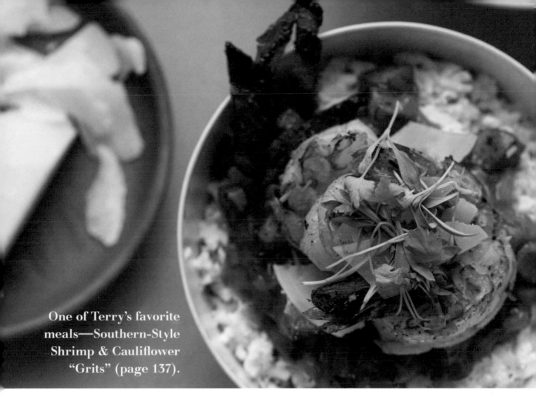

One of Terry's favorite meals—Southern-Style Shrimp & Cauliflower "Grits" (page 137).

The Zesty Coconut Lime Skirt Steak & Barley Fried "Rice" (page 163) is a legitimate crowd-pleaser. Make it for your family or a dinner with friends!

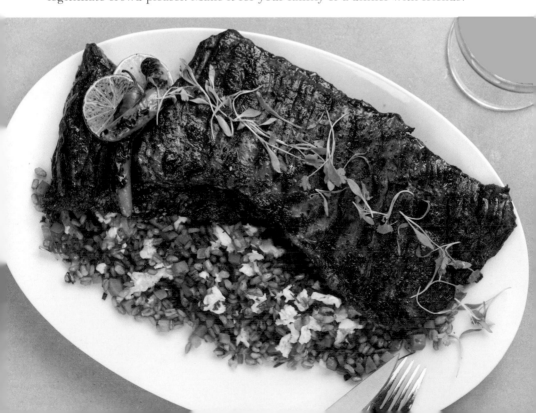

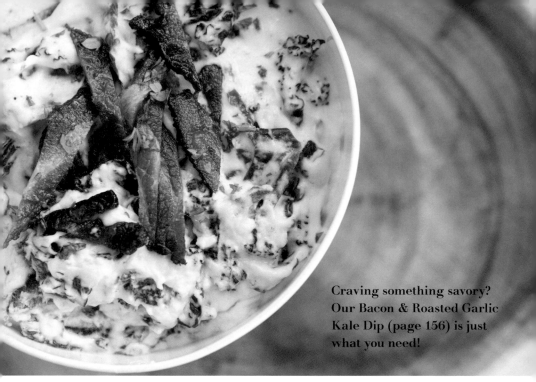

Craving something savory? Our Bacon & Roasted Garlic Kale Dip (page 156) is just what you need!

So many tasty choices! Fat Bomb Burger Sliders (page 121), Loaded Celery Sticks (page 120), and Roasted Cauliflower Hummus (page 114) are ready to be enjoyed.

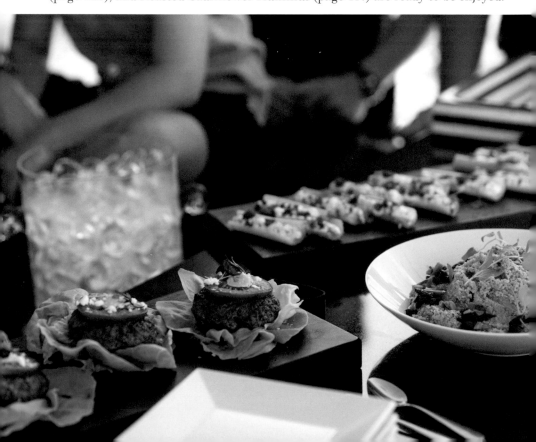

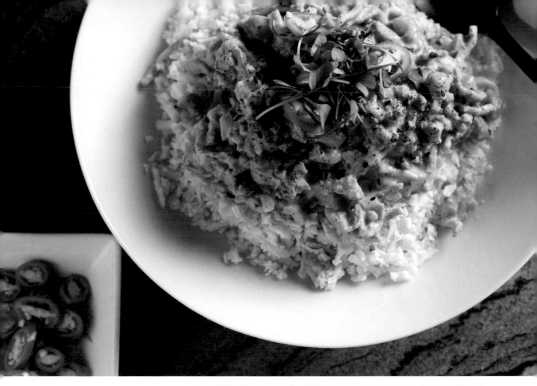

This White Turkey
Chili over Cauliflower
Cilantro "Rice"
(page 167) is perfect for
family dinner night,
or for when you
want really amazing
leftovers the next day.

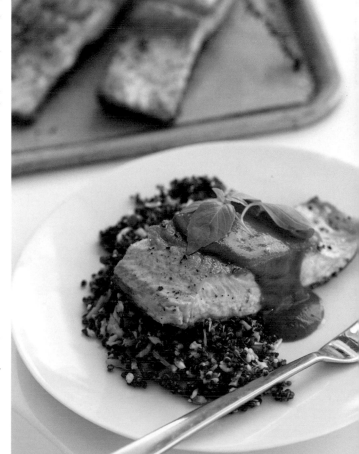

Treat yourself with our
Herb & Tomato Salmon
with Quinoa Pilaf
(page 173)!

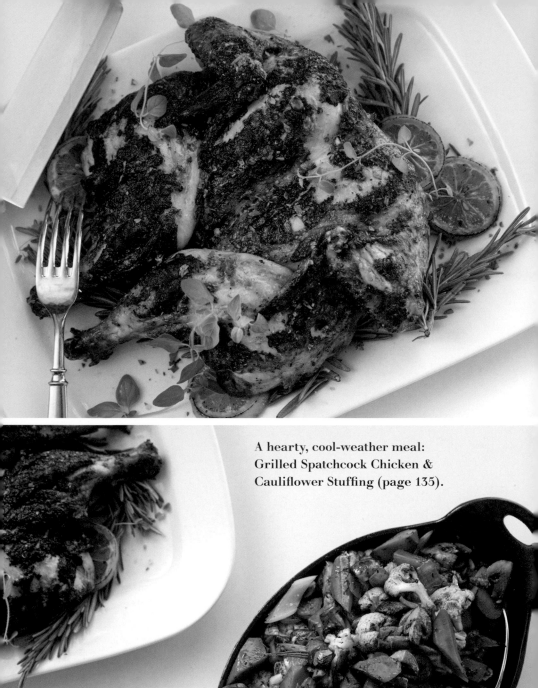

A hearty, cool-weather meal: Grilled Spatchcock Chicken & Cauliflower Stuffing (page 135).

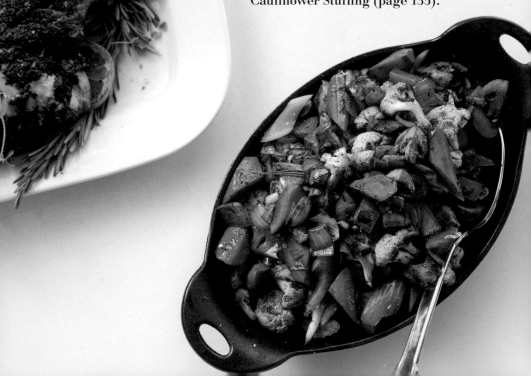

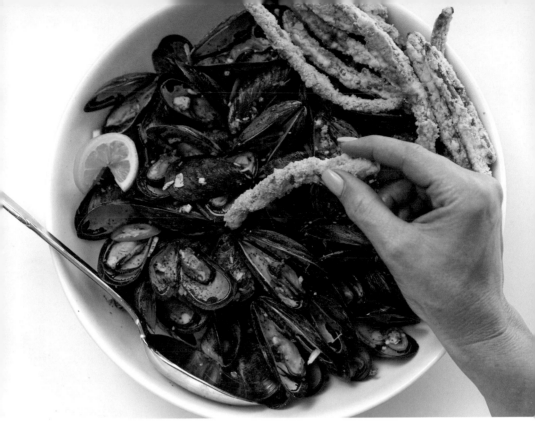

Dipping into some spicy mussels, which pair perfectly with our green bean "fries" (page 171).

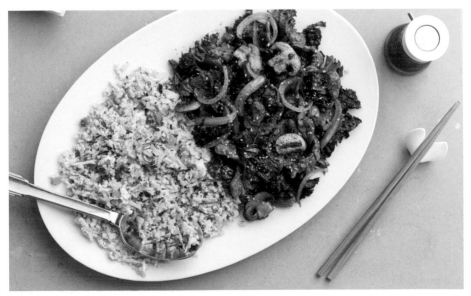

Craving takeout? Make this DKFD-approved Beef & Kale Teriyaki with Cauliflower Fried "Rice" (page 161) instead; it's better tasting and better for you!

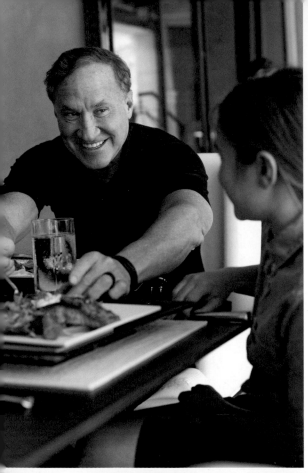

Teaching our kids how to live the yummiest and healthiest lifestyle!

We love eating family style! It's not always easy to get everyone to the table, but when we do it's our favorite time.

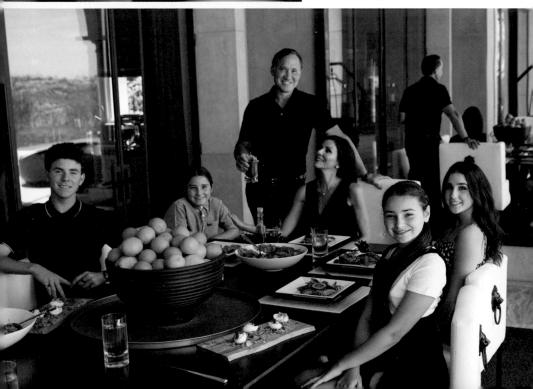

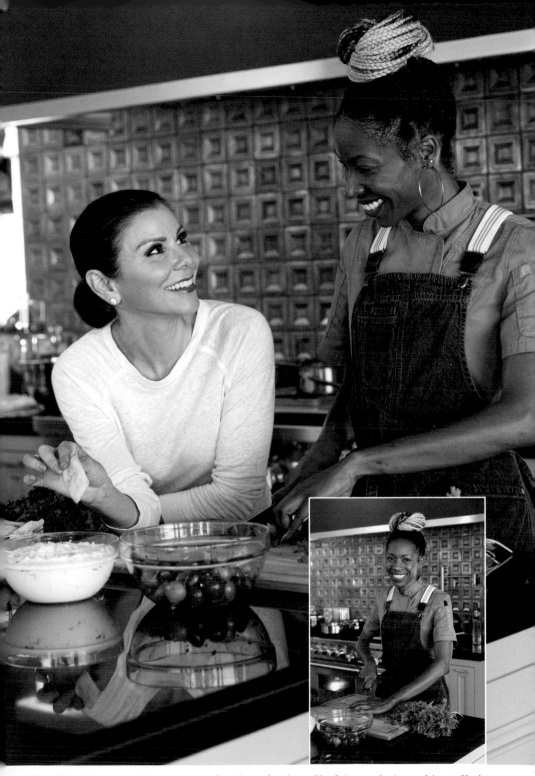

Yes, I'm always sneaking a bite (or three!) when Chef Amanda is cooking! She's great at making incredibly flavorful, healthy dishes for the whole family.

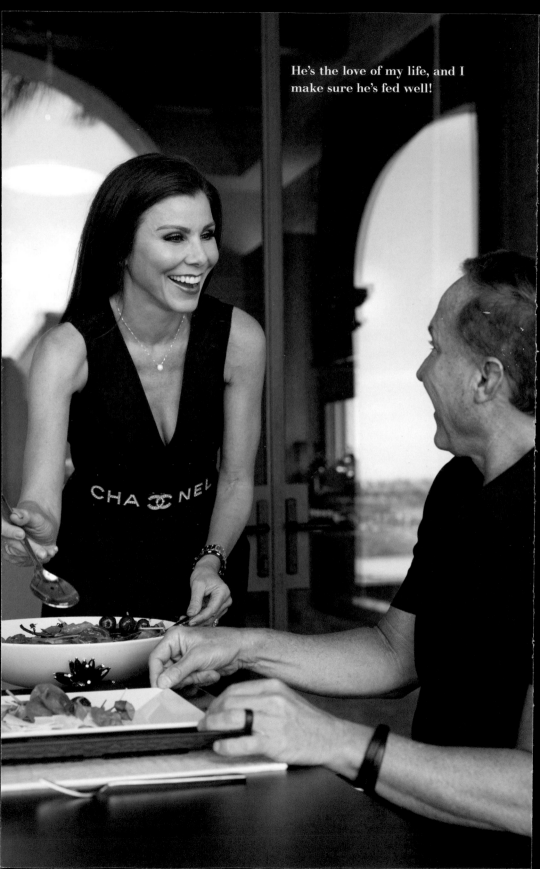

He's the love of my life, and I make sure he's fed well!

Red Wine Vinaigrette

Grab yourself a few 2-ounce containers to prep this dressing for quick on-the-go access when you're meal-prepping for the week.

MAKES A LITTLE LESS THAN 1 CUP

1 teaspoon Dijon mustard

1 teaspoon fresh lemon juice

1 teaspoon garlic powder

1 teaspoon onion powder

1 teaspoon erythritol

1 teaspoon sea salt

$1/2$ teaspoon dried rosemary

$1/2$ teaspoon dried thyme

$1/2$ teaspoon ground black pepper

$1/4$ cup red wine vinegar

2 tablespoons water

$1/2$ cup olive oil

In a blender, mix all the ingredients except for the olive oil. With the machine running, slowly pour in the olive oil in a steady stream to emulsify. Store in a glass container in the refrigerator.

White Wine Vinaigrette

This is one of Terry's favorite dressings! He loves pairing it with fresh salads like our arugula (page 131) or spinach (page 133) offerings.

MAKES A LITTLE LESS THAN 1 CUP

1 teaspoon Dijon mustard

1 teaspoon fresh lemon juice

1 teaspoon garlic powder

1 teaspoon onion powder

1 teaspoon erythritol

1 teaspoon sea salt

1/2 teaspoon dried rosemary

1/2 teaspoon dried thyme

1/2 teaspoon ground black pepper

2 tablespoons water

1/4 cup white wine vinegar

1/2 cup olive oil

In a blender, mix all the ingredients except for the olive oil. With the machine running, slowly pour in the olive oil in a steady stream to emulsify. Store in a glass container in the refrigerator.

Asian-Style Vinaigrette

One of Kat's (the Dubrows' middle daughter) favorite things is an Asian-style chopped chicken salad. For a DKFD version, prepare a Pan-Roasted Chicken Breast (page 183), chop it, and toss it with this dressing and our Bok Choy Salad (page 141).

MAKES A LITTLE LESS THAN 1 CUP

1 teaspoon Dijon mustard

1 teaspoon lemon juice

1 teaspoon garlic powder

1 teaspoon ground ginger

1 teaspoon erythritol

¼ cup rice vinegar

2 tablespoons liquid aminos

1 tablespoon sesame oil

½ cup olive oil

In a blender, mix all the ingredients except for the sesame oil and olive oil. With the machine running, slowly pour in the oils in a steady stream to emulsify. Store in a glass container in the refrigerator.

Refuel Recipes

(4-Hour Window)

Rosemary & Cracked Black Pepper Crackers

This is one of our favorite recipes for entertaining! Everyone loves crackers, but they can be really high in carbs. Pair these with the Bruschetta Topping & Herbed Cottage Cheese (page 157) for a fabulous snack or appetizer.

SERVES 6

2 cups super-fine almond flour

2 teaspoons finely chopped fresh rosemary

2 teaspoons cracked black pepper

1/2 teaspoon sea salt

2 large cage-free eggs

2 to 4 tablespoons ice water

Olive oil

1. Preheat the oven to 350°F. Line a baking sheet with parchment paper.

2. In a food processor, pulse together the almond flour, rosemary, pepper, and salt until well combined.

3. Pulse in the eggs and 2 tablespoons of the ice water. The dough should be crumbly but pliable. Add more water if the dough will not stay together.

4. Oil your hands and place the dough ball between two sheets of parchment paper. Evenly roll the dough to 1/8 inch thick. Cut out 3¾ × 1½-inch rectangular crackers and place them on the prepared baking sheet. Gather the dough scraps, reroll, and cut out more crackers. If desired, lightly prick a fork just into the tops of the crackers in a uniform design.

5. Bake the crackers until golden brown and somewhat crisp, 8 to 12 minutes, rotating the pan front to back halfway through the cooking time.

6. Let cool on the pan until safe to handle, then transfer carefully to a wire rack to cool completely and crisp more, at least 15 to 20 minutes, before serving.

Bacon & Roasted Garlic Kale Dip

This high-fat dip is a craving killer! It's definitely best when served warm, and goes great with our Rosemary & Cracked Black Pepper Crackers (page 155). For extra flavor, consider adding a dollop of this to a breakfast burger.

SERVES 8

2 tablespoons olive oil

2 tablespoons minced shallots

5 cloves roasted garlic, minced (page 146)

1 bunch kale, stems and midribs removed, leaves chopped

3/4 cup Keto Bone Broth (page 147) or water

1 cup plain whole-milk Greek yogurt

1/2 cup shredded mozzarella cheese

2 tablespoons shaved parmesan cheese

4 slices uncured bacon, cooked and sliced or crumbled

1/2 teaspoon salt

1/4 teaspoon ground black pepper

1. In a large nonstick skillet, heat the oil over medium-high heat. Add the shallots, garlic, and kale. Sauté for 1 to 2 minutes, then add the broth. Cover and cook, stirring occasionally, until the vegetables are tender and the broth is evaporated, another 2 minutes.

2. Reduce the heat to medium-low and add the yogurt, stirring until well incorporated. Stir in the mozzarella, 1 tablespoon of the parmesan, and the bacon pieces, reserving some for garnish. Finish with salt and pepper.

3. Transfer to a serving dish and top with the reserved bacon and the remaining 1 tablespoon parmesan. (Optional: Transfer the mixture to a broilerproof dish and broil in the oven for 30 seconds to 1 minute or until the cheese on top begins to brown and bubble.)

Bruschetta Topping & Herbed Cottage Cheese

Although you can have this dish at any time of year thanks to modern farming practices, it is truly at its best during tomato season, which is typically from May to October (specific dates depend on where you live). Heather and Terry especially love end-of-summer heirloom tomatoes; they're naturally sweet and so very beautiful. Enjoy with our Rosemary & Cracked Black Pepper Crackers (page 155).

SERVES 4

1 cup halved or quartered (depending on size) cherry tomatoes

2 teaspoons minced shallots

1 teaspoon grated lemon zest

2 teaspoons fresh lemon juice

1 tablespoon olive oil

1 teaspoon sea salt

$1/2$ teaspoon ground black pepper

3 tablespoons chopped fresh basil

1 cup whole-milk cottage cheese

1 tablespoon chopped fresh parsley

$1/4$ cup grated parmesan cheese

1. Chill a serving bowl in the freezer.

2. In a nonreactive bowl, toss together the tomatoes, shallots, lemon zest, lemon juice, olive oil, salt, pepper, and 2 tablespoons of the basil. Mix well to incorporate all the ingredients. Set aside.

3. In a small bowl, combine the cottage cheese, parsley, parmesan, and remaining 1 tablespoon basil.

4. Put the herbed cottage cheese in the chilled serving bowl and top with the tomato mixture.

Spicy Kale & Brazil Nut Dip

This spicy dip is zesty and colorful! Step up the presentation by adding some more color with radish sprouts.

SERVES 5

1 bunch Tuscan kale, stems and midribs removed

³/₄ cup Keto Bone Broth (page 147)

2 jalapeños, seeded

2 teaspoons minced shallot

1 cup Brazil nuts, toasted

¹/₄ cup fresh cilantro

¹/₂ cup avocado oil mayonnaise

³/₄ teaspoon La Baleine Kosher Sea Salt

1. In a medium saucepan, combine the kale and bone broth. Heat over medium-high heat, cover, and simmer until the kale is tender, about 4 minutes. Drain the kale and transfer it to a food processor.

2. Add the jalapeños, shallot, nuts, cilantro, mayonnaise, and salt. Puree until smooth. Serve chilled or at room temperature.

Avocado Hummus

Hummus is a family favorite, and this avocado-based one is a Coco (the Dubrows' youngest daughter) favorite! Enjoy this flavor-packed dip with Crispy Okra Chips (page 115) or Killer Kale Chips (page 117).

SERVES 6

2 avocados, halved and pitted

$\frac{1}{2}$ cup tahini

$\frac{1}{4}$ cup hulled sunflower seeds

1 teaspoon minced shallot

$\frac{1}{2}$ teaspoon fresh lemon juice

$\frac{1}{2}$ cup loosely packed cilantro sprigs

1 teaspoon La Baleine Kosher Sea Salt

$\frac{1}{2}$ teaspoon ground cumin

$\frac{1}{2}$ teaspoon ground black pepper

$\frac{1}{2}$ cup olive oil

1. Scoop the avocado flesh into a food processor. Add the tahini, sunflower seeds, shallot, lemon juice, cilantro, salt, cumin, and pepper. Puree until well blended.

2. With the machine running, stream in the oil and continue blending until smooth. Add water if necessary to loosen the consistency. Serve immediately or refrigerate.

Billion Dollar Dip

A remixed, DKFD-friendly version of the famous Neiman Marcus dip (referred to as "Million Dollar Dip"). Serve the dip with our Rosemary & Cracked Black Pepper Crackers (page 155).

SERVES 6

1½ cups avocado oil mayonnaise

½ cup slivered almonds

½ cup uncured bacon, cooked and crumbled (from 8 slices)

½ cup shredded mozzarella cheese

½ cup shredded parmesan cheese

2 green onions (green parts only), chopped

½ tablespoon chopped fresh parsley

½ tablespoon chopped fresh basil

1 teaspoon minced shallot

½ teaspoon ground black pepper

In a large bowl, combine all the ingredients, using a spatula to incorporate them well. Serve immediately.

Beef & Kale Teriyaki with Cauliflower Fried "Rice"

Terry loves Asian fusion dishes! The family enjoys some sort of stir-fry at least once a week, and this beef and kale teriyaki is also a hit with the kids!

SERVES 4

Marinated Beef

2 tablespoons tamari

1 tablespoon brown sugar replacement

2 garlic cloves, minced

1 tablespoon minced fresh ginger

1½ pounds grass-fed beef sirloin steak, cut into wide strips

Cauliflower Fried "Rice"

1 medium head cauliflower, trimmed

2 tablespoons ghee

¼ cup chopped carrots

½ cup chopped onions

2 large cage-free eggs, scrambled and chopped

2 tablespoons chopped green onion (green parts only)

½ tablespoon sesame seeds

2 tablespoons tamari or liquid aminos

1 teaspoon sesame oil

To Finish

2 tablespoons avocado oil

10 button mushrooms, sliced

½ bunch red kale, stems and midribs removed, cut into wide strips

1 teaspoon sesame oil

½ teaspoon La Baleine Kosher Sea Salt

1. Marinate the beef: In a medium bowl, whisk together the tamari, brown sugar replacement, garlic, and ginger. Add the sliced beef and cover with plastic wrap. Set aside to marinate for a minimum of 1 hour.

2. Meanwhile, prepare the cauliflower fried "rice:" Rice the cauli-

flower in a food processor with the grating disc or grate by hand. Set the riced cauliflower aside.

3. In a large nonstick skillet or wok, melt the ghee over medium-high heat. Add the carrots and onions and sauté until tender, 3 to 4 minutes. Add the scrambled eggs, green onions, and sesame seeds. Toss until all the ingredients are well incorporated. Add the riced cauliflower, tamari, and sesame oil and toss to incorporate. Transfer to a serving dish and keep warm while you finish the teriyaki.

4. To finish: Using the same pan or wok, heat the avocado oil over medium-high heat. Add the mushrooms and cook until caramelized or golden brown, 2 to 3 minutes.

5. Reserving the marinade, remove the steak and add it to the pan to sear for 1 to 2 minutes on each side. (If increasing the recipe, you may have to work in batches.) Add the marinade and cook the steak and mushrooms until the marinade is reduced by one quarter, about 2 minutes. Add the kale and cook for 1 minute more. Stir in the sesame oil and salt.

6. Serve the beef and kale over the fried "rice" and enjoy!

Zesty Coconut Lime Skirt Steak & Barley Fried "Rice"

This fun dish is great for a cookout or a perfect-grilling-weather sort of afternoon. Nicky (the Dubrows' son) especially loves a juicy and flavor-packed steak! Add some complexity to your steak by incorporating mesquite wood chips!

SERVES 4

Marinated Skirt Steak

1/2 cup coconut oil, melted

1 tablespoon minced fresh ginger

2 garlic cloves, minced

2 teaspoons grated lime zest

2 tablespoons fresh lime juice

1 teaspoon chili powder

1/2 teaspoon ground cloves

11/2 pounds grass-fed skirt steak

Barley Fried "Rice"

2 tablespoons ghee

1/4 cup chopped carrots

1/2 cup chopped onions

2 large cage-free eggs, scrambled and chopped

2 tablespoons chopped green onion (greens parts only)

1/2 tablespoon sesame seeds

2 cups cooked barley

2 tablespoons tamari or liquid aminos

1 teaspoon sesame oil

To Finish

1 teaspoon La Baleine Kosher Sea Salt

1/2 teaspoon ground black pepper

1. Marinate the skirt steak: In a large bowl, whisk together the coconut oil, ginger, garlic, lime zest, lime juice, chili powder, and cloves. Add the steak and be sure to toss and massage it well with marinade. Cover with plastic wrap and set aside for a minimum of 1 hour.

2. Preheat a grill to medium-high heat.

3. Meanwhile, prepare the barley fried "rice:" In large nonstick skil-

let or wok, melt the ghee over medium-high heat. Add the carrots and onions and sauté until tender, 2 to 3 minutes. Add the scrambled eggs, green onion, and sesame seeds. Toss until all the ingredients are well incorporated. Add the barley, tamari, and sesame oil and toss to incorporate. Transfer to a serving dish and keep warm.

4. Reserving the marinade, remove the steak and rub it down to evenly distribute the marinade and also remove any excess coconut oil that could flare up. Salt and pepper the steak and add it to the grill. Sear the steak over direct heat for 2 minutes on each side. Move the steak to indirect heat, close the grill, and cook for 6 to 8 minutes for medium, or until desired level of doneness is achieved.

5. Move the beef back over direct heat and baste with some of the reserved marinade and grill for another 2 to 3 minutes. Allow the beef to rest for about 5 minutes before slicing.

6. Serve the steak over barley fried "rice" and enjoy!

Grilled Flank Steak with Garden Vegetable Ratatouille

Rare steak is one of Heather's favorite things to eat, and this is definitely a meal fit for a queen! Be sure not to skip the marinating step—that's the secret to this dish being excellent.

SERVES 4

Marinated Flank Steak

2 tablespoons tamari

¼ cup olive oil

2 tablespoons Dijon mustard

2 tablespoons fresh lemon juice

2 tablespoons red wine vinegar

1 tablespoon dried thyme

2 garlic cloves, minced

½ teaspoon ground black pepper

1½ pounds flank steak

Garden Vegetable Ratatouille

2 tablespoons olive oil

2 shallots, sliced

1 small to medium eggplant, diced

3 garlic cloves, minced

1 green bell pepper, cut into large squares

1 medium zucchini, cut into large dice

2 Roma (plum) tomatoes, diced

¼ cup chopped basil leaves

¼ cup Keto Bone Broth (page 147)

1 teaspoon sea salt

½ teaspoon ground black pepper

To Finish

Cooking spray

1 teaspoon sea salt

1. Marinate the flank steak: In a small bowl, whisk together the tamari, ¼ cup olive oil, mustard, lemon juice, vinegar, thyme, garlic, and black pepper. Place the meat in a zip-seal bag, pour the marinade over the steak, and seal. Allow steak to marinate for at least 2 hours.

2. Meanwhile, make the ratatouille: In a large nonstick skillet, heat the 2 tablespoons olive oil over medium heat. Add the shallots and sauté until translucent, 2 to 3 minutes. Add the eggplant and cook

until just fork-tender, another 2 to 3 minutes. Add the garlic, bell pepper, zucchini, and tomatoes and cook on medium-high heat until the zucchini is fork-tender. Stir in the basil and bone broth. Once the broth has reduced almost completely and resembles a thickened sauce, add the salt and pepper. Set aside and keep warm.

3. To finish: Preheat a grill to medium-high.

4. Remove the flank steak from the marinade and pat dry with paper towels. Lightly coat both sides of the steak with cooking spray and sprinkle with the salt.

5. Grill over direct heat for 4 to 6 minutes per side for a crispy sear and medium-rare doneness, or until the internal temperature reaches 135°F. Or continue cooking over indirect heat to reach desired doneness.

6. Allow the steak to rest for at least 5 minutes. Slice the steak against the grain with the knife at an angle to the cutting board. Serve alongside the ratatouille.

White Turkey Chili over Cauliflower Cilantro "Rice"

Cooler California days call for something that warms the soul (without overdoing it on the carbs!). This chili does just that. Add ancho chili powder for extra heat and a smoky flavor.

SERVES 5 OR 6

2 tablespoons coconut oil

½ medium onion, diced

1 shallot, diced

2 jalapeños, seeded and finely diced

1 pound ground turkey

½ tablespoon ground coriander

½ tablespoon ground cumin

2 teaspoons sea salt

1 teaspoon celery salt

1 teaspoon garlic powder

1 teaspoon ground white pepper

1 (15.5-ounce) can chickpeas, drained and rinsed

2 cups heavy (whipping) cream

1 tablespoon Dijon mustard

2 tablespoons chopped fresh cilantro, plus more for serving

Chili powder, for serving

Cauliflower Cilantro "Rice"

1 medium head cauliflower, trimmed

2 tablespoons ghee

1 teaspoon sea salt

2 tablespoons finely chopped fresh cilantro

1. In a large pot or Dutch oven, heat the coconut oil over medium heat. Add the onion, shallot, and jalapeños and cook until translucent, 1 to 2 minutes. Increase the heat to medium-high, add the ground turkey, and sprinkle with the coriander, cumin, sea salt, celery salt, garlic powder, and white pepper. Cook the turkey until browned and crumbled, 10 to 12 minutes, breaking it up with a spatula as it cooks.

2. Add the chickpeas, cream, and mustard. Bring to a simmer and cook the chili for 5 minutes, stirring often. Reduce the heat, stir in the cilantro, and keep warm.

3. Make the cauliflower rice: Rice the cauliflower in a food processor with the grating disc or grate by hand.

4. In a large nonstick skillet, melt the ghee over medium-high heat. Add the cauliflower rice, sea salt, and cilantro and toss together. Sauté, tossing gently, for 2 minutes.

5. To serve, spoon the cauliflower rice into individual serving bowls and ladle chili over them. Garnish with cilantro and chili powder.

Grilled Chicken Thighs with Buttered Broccoli

These grilled chicken thighs are so juicy and delicious! Be sure to watch for flames that arise from the melting chicken fat. If flames do appear, adjust the flame or the position of the grill accordingly.

SERVES 6

4 tablespoons olive oil

Grated zest and juice of 1 lemon

1/2 tablespoon chopped fresh rosemary

3/4 teaspoon chopped fresh thyme

2 teaspoons paprika

2 teaspoons ground black pepper

1 teaspoon garlic powder

1 teaspoon onion powder

6 bone-in, skin-on chicken thighs

1 1/2 tablespoons La Baleine Kosher Sea Salt

Buttered Broccoli

8 tablespoons ghee

2 pounds broccoli, cut into florets

2 tablespoons chopped fresh chives

1 teaspoon La Baleine Kosher Sea Salt

1/2 teaspoon ground black pepper

1. Preheat a grill to a medium-high.

2. In a small bowl, mix together the olive oil, lemon zest, lemon juice, rosemary, thyme, paprika, pepper, garlic powder, and onion powder. Brush the chicken all over with the seasoned olive oil.

3. When ready to grill, season the chicken all over with the salt. Place the chicken on the grill, skin-side down over direct heat, and close the grill. Cook until the skin begins to render fat and become crispy, 8 to 10 minutes, rotating the chicken halfway through cooking, then reduce the heat to maintain a temperature of 325°F. Turn the chicken over, close the grill, and cook for another 8 to 10 minutes on each side or until the internal temperature reaches 165°F.

4. Meanwhile, make the broccoli: In a large nonstick skillet, melt the ghee over medium-high heat. Add the broccoli and cook until it begins to brown, about 5 minutes. Add the chives, salt, and pepper and sauté, tossing lightly to incorporate flavors, until the chives become fragrant, 1 minute. Keep warm.

5. Remove the chicken thighs from the grill and serve alongside the buttered broccoli.

Spicy Mussels & Green Bean "Fries"

This DKFD-friendly version of moules-frites (mussels + French fries) brings restaurant-quality cooking straight to your home! When plating, make sure to also serve the sauce. It's great for the mussels and it's a-m-a-z-i-n-g for dunking the green bean "fries."

SERVES 4

Green Bean "Fries"

⅔ cup grated parmesan cheese

½ teaspoon paprika

½ teaspoon garlic powder

½ teaspoon onion powder

½ teaspoon Himalayan pink salt

¼ teaspoon ground black pepper

1 large cage-free egg

12 ounces green beans, rinsed, dried, and ends snipped

Spicy Mussels

2 tablespoons avocado oil

1 tablespoon chopped shallots

2 garlic cloves, minced

2 serrano peppers, seeded and cut into rings

½ cup Keto Bone Broth (page 147)

2 tablespoons grass-fed unsalted butter

1 teaspoon grated lime zest

1½ pounds mussels, cleaned and rinsed

2 tablespoons chopped fresh parsley

2 teaspoons La Baleine Kosher Sea Salt

1 teaspoon ground black pepper

1. Make the green bean "fries": Preheat the oven to 400°F. Line a baking sheet with foil.

2. On a wide shallow plate, use a fork to blend the parmesan, paprika, garlic powder, onion powder, pink salt, and pepper.

3. In a large bowl, lightly beat the egg. Add the green beans and toss to coat evenly. Working in batches, coat the green beans in the cheese mixture, tossing and sprinkling the cheese to cover evenly. Arrange the beans on the baking sheet.

4. Bake until the green beans are golden brown, 10 to 12 minutes. Remove from the oven and keep warm.

5. Meanwhile, prepare the mussels: In a large skillet, heat the avocado over medium-high heat. Add the shallots, garlic, and serranos and sauté until the shallots are translucent and the garlic is fragrant, 2 to 3 minutes. Add the broth, butter, and lime zest to the pan and cook for another 2 to 3 minutes to build the flavor in the broth.

6. Add the mussels and tightly cover the pan. Cook the mussels until they've all opened, 2 to 3 minutes. Throw out any unopened mussels. Toss with the parsley, salt, and pepper.

7. Serve in a bowl with the broth and the green bean fries alongside.

Herb & Tomato Salmon with Quinoa Pilaf

Coco absolutely adores wild-caught salmon! This dish is really great for busy weeknights, and pairs well with a quick pot of pasta (for kids or for you on your cheat day!).

SERVES 2

Quinoa Pilaf

1 tablespoon ghee

2 tablespoons chopped carrots

2 tablespoons chopped celery

¼ cup chopped onion

1 cup cooked quinoa (cooked according to package directions)

Herb & Tomato Salmon

2 ounces pancetta, diced

1 teaspoon olive oil (optional)

2 skin-on wild-caught salmon fillets (4 ounces each), at room temperature

1 teaspoon sea salt

½ teaspoon ground black pepper

2 tablespoons minced shallots

1 garlic clove, minced

2 tablespoons dry white wine

2 tablespoons Keto Bone Broth (page 147)

1 teaspoon grated lemon zest

1 tablespoon tomato paste

⅓ cup heavy (whipping) cream

2 tablespoons chopped fresh basil

½ tablespoon grass-fed unsalted butter

1. Make the quinoa pilaf: In a large nonstick skillet, melt the ghee over medium-high heat. Add the carrots and celery and sauté until fragrant, 2 to 3 minutes. Add the onions and sauté until they are translucent, 2 to 3 minutes. Add the quinoa and toss all the ingredients to incorporate well. Remove from the heat and keep warm.

2. Make the salmon: In a medium skillet, cook the pancetta over medium-low heat to slowly render the fat. When the pancetta is crispy, remove the crisped pieces and leave the fat in the pan.

3. Drain all but 2 tablespoons of fat from the skillet. (If there isn't enough fat, add the olive oil.) Increase the heat to medium-high. Season both sides of the salmon with the salt and pepper. Add to the pan skin-side down and sear undisturbed for 3 to 4 minutes. Flip the fillets with a fish spatula and continue cooking until the salmon is opaque and somewhat flaky, 4 to 5 minutes. Set the salmon aside and keep warm.

4. Return the skillet to medium heat and add the shallots and garlic, sautéing them until translucent, 1 to 2 minutes. Add the wine, broth, and lemon zest and allow to reduce halfway. Stir in the tomato paste and cream. Bring to a simmer to thicken the sauce. Stir in the basil, butter, and pancetta.

5. Plate the quinoa pilaf and salmon on individual serving plates and spoon sauce over them. Enjoy immediately.

BBQ Shrimp with Walnut Broccolini

Heather and Terry both love textured dishes with crunch! Adding walnuts to a dish like this not only gives it a little bit of fun, but increases the fat, protein, and crunch, too.

SERVES 6

Walnut Broccolini

Cooking spray

4 bunches broccolini, stems trimmed

2 tablespoons walnut oil

3 tablespoons tamari or liquid aminos

$\frac{1}{2}$ teaspoon ground ginger

$\frac{1}{2}$ teaspoon red pepper flakes

2 teaspoons monk fruit sweetener

2 garlic cloves, minced

$\frac{1}{2}$ cup walnut pieces

BBQ Shrimp

$\frac{1}{2}$ teaspoon sea salt

$\frac{1}{4}$ teaspoon dried oregano

$\frac{1}{4}$ teaspoon dried thyme

$\frac{1}{4}$ teaspoon paprika

$\frac{1}{4}$ teaspoon garlic powder

$\frac{1}{4}$ teaspoon onion powder

$\frac{1}{4}$ teaspoon red pepper flakes

$\frac{1}{4}$ teaspoon ground black pepper

$\frac{1}{4}$ teaspoon cayenne pepper

$1\frac{1}{2}$ pounds wild-caught shrimp, peeled and deveined

2 tablespoons olive oil

2 tablespoons Keto Bone Broth (page 147) or water

2 tablespoons Ketchup (page 148)

2 teaspoons Dijon mustard

2 teaspoons apple cider vinegar

2 teaspoons Worcestershire sauce

1 tablespoon chopped fresh cilantro

1. Prepare the broccolini: Preheat the oven to 375°F. Lightly coat a rimmed baking sheet with cooking spray.

2. In a medium bowl, toss the broccolini with the walnut oil, tamari, ginger, pepper flakes, and sweetener. Spread on the baking sheet.

3. Transfer to the oven and bake until just fork-tender, 10 to 12 minutes. Remove from the oven and toss the broccolini with the garlic and walnuts. Return to the oven and bake until the garlic is fra-

grant but not burning, 2 to 3 minutes. Remove from the oven and keep warm.

4. Make the BBQ shrimp: In a small bowl, mix together the sea salt, oregano, thyme, paprika, garlic powder, onion powder, pepper flakes, black pepper, and cayenne. Season the shrimp evenly with the spice mixture.

5. In a large nonstick skillet, heat the olive oil over medium-high heat. Add the shrimp and sear 1 to 2 minutes on each side depending on their size. Add the broth, ketchup, mustard, vinegar, and Worcestershire and stir well. Finish with the cilantro.

6. Serve the shrimp over the broccolini.

Parmesan-Crusted Cod with "Invisible Rice" Pilaf

While this is an easy weeknight dish that is great for the whole family, traditionally prepared white rice isn't ideal for the DKFD. However, when you prepare the rice as directed here, you make it a perfect side dish for the Refuel window!

SERVES 4

"Invisible Rice"

1 teaspoon salt

1 teaspoon coconut oil

1 cup long-grain rice

Parmesan-Crusted Cod

$^3/_4$ cup grated parmesan cheese

2 teaspoons paprika

$^1/_2$ teaspoon garlic powder

$^1/_2$ teaspoon onion powder

1 teaspoon La Baleine Kosher Sea Salt

$^1/_2$ teaspoon ground black pepper

1 tablespoon chopped fresh parsley

1 teaspoon fresh lemon juice

4 cod fillets (6 ounces each)

1 tablespoon olive oil

For the Pilaf

1 tablespoon ghee

2 tablespoons chopped carrot

Lemon slices, for serving

2 tablespoons chopped celery

$^1/_4$ cup chopped onion

1. Make the "Invisible Rice": In a saucepan, bring 2 cups of water to a boil. Add the salt and coconut oil. Stir in the rice, cover, and simmer for 40 minutes. Transfer the cooked rice to a container to cool to room temperature, then refrigerate the rice for at least 12 hours before using.

2. Cook the cod: Preheat the oven to 400°F. Line a baking sheet with foil.

3. In a shallow bowl, mix together the parmesan, paprika, garlic powder, onion powder, salt, pepper, parsley, and lemon juice.

4. Coat the cod fillets evenly with the olive oil. Dip each of the cod fillets into the parmesan mixture. Use your fingers to press the coating lightly into the fillets. Transfer the cod to the lined baking sheet. Bake until the fish is opaque and flaky, 10 to 15 minutes.

5. Meanwhile, prepare the pilaf: In a large nonstick skillet, melt the ghee over medium-high heat. Add the carrots and celery and cook until fragrant, 2 to 3 minutes. Add the onion and cook until the onion is translucent, 2 to 3 minutes. Add the chilled "invisible rice" and toss all the ingredients with a fork to incorporate. Increase the heat to high and add 2 tablespoons of water to steam the rice thoroughly. Cook until the rice is heated all the way through, 45 seconds to 1 minute.

6. Serve the pilaf alongside the cod with sliced lemons.

Spaghetti Squash with Parmesan & Pine Nuts

You might have seen other recipes that use steaming or microwaving to prepare spaghetti squash, but taking the time to roast it will reward you with richer squash that's less watery than other preparations.

Pair this with any of our Perfectly Pan-Roasted Proteins, like wild-caught salmon (page 185)!

SERVES 4

2 tablespoons olive oil

1 medium spaghetti squash, halved and seeded

2 teaspoons sea salt

1/2 teaspoon coarsely ground black pepper

2 teaspoons chopped shallots

2 teaspoons White Wine Vinaigrette (page 150)

1/4 cup finely chopped fresh parsley

2 tablespoons finely chopped fresh chives

3/4 cup freshly grated parmesan cheese

1/4 cup pine nuts, toasted

1. Preheat the oven to 375°F. Line a rimmed baking sheet with aluminum foil and place an oven-safe wire rack on top of it.

2. Rub 1½ tablespoons of the oil all over the squash. Season the insides with 1 teaspoon of the salt and the pepper.

3. Place the seasoned squash cut-sides down atop the wire rack and roast it in the oven until fork-tender, 25 to 30 minutes.

4. Remove the squash from the oven and set aside until cool enough to handle, at least 10 minutes. Scrape out the insides with a fork and let them stand in a paper towel–lined colander. Gently squeeze a few times to release any excess water.

5. Meanwhile, heat the remaining olive oil in a large skillet over medium heat. Add the shallots and cook until fragrant and translucent, 1 to 2 minutes.

6. Increase the heat to medium-high and add the spaghetti squash, vinaigrette, herbs, and remaining salt. Sauté for 1 to 2 more minutes to heat the ingredients thoroughly.

7. Remove the skillet from the heat and stir in the parmesan. Top with toasted pine nuts and enjoy!

Brown Rice Pilaf

Serve this with any of our Perfectly Pan-Roasted Proteins, like chicken breasts (page 183) or wild-caught salmon (page 185).

SERVES 2

1 tablespoon ghee

2 tablespoons chopped carrots

2 tablespoons chopped celery

¼ cup chopped onion

1 cup cooked brown rice (cooked according to package directions)

1. In a large nonstick skillet, melt the ghee over medium-high heat. Add the carrots and celery and sauté until fragrant, 2 to 3 minutes.

2. Add the onion and sauté until the onions are translucent, 2 to 3 minutes.

3. Add the cooked brown rice and toss all the ingredients with a fork to incorporate them well.

4. Increase the heat to high and add 2 tablespoons of water to steam the rice thoroughly. Cook until the rice is heated all the way through, 45 seconds to 1 minute.

Perfectly Pan-Roasted Proteins:
Rib Eyes

Make a perfect steak every single time with this recipe! Feel free to pull this recipe out for date night and special occasions, too.

SERVES 2

2 tablespoons grapeseed oil

2 rib-eye steaks

1 teaspoon sea salt

1/2 teaspoon ground black pepper

2 tablespoons grass-fed unsalted butter

1/4 shallot, sliced

4 sprigs fresh thyme

1 garlic clove, smashed

1. Allow the steaks to sit out for 25 to 30 minutes to come to room temperature.

2. In a large cast-iron skillet, heat the grapeseed oil over medium-high heat. Season the steaks with salt and pepper and cook until well-seared or browned on the outside, 5 to 6 minutes. Flip the steaks frequently to achieve even cooking. (For a more well-done steak, transfer to a 400°F oven and cook for 8 to 12 minutes depending on desired doneness.)

3. Add the butter, shallot, thyme, and garlic to the pan and cook, basting the steaks, until the butter begins to foam, 2 to 3 minutes.

4. Remove the skillet from the heat and let the steaks rest for 3 to 4 minutes before serving. Serve drizzled with butter from the pan.

Perfectly Pan-Roasted Proteins: Chicken Breasts

This recipe is quick and easy, and makes chicken breasts that pair well with most any side item featured in the recipes, such as Brown Rice Pilaf (page 181). You can double this recipe and chop the chicken to prepare for a week's worth of lunches.

SERVES 2

2 boneless, skinless chicken breasts

2 tablespoons grapeseed oil

1 teaspoon sea salt

$1/2$ teaspoon ground black pepper

2 tablespoons grass-fed unsalted butter

4 sprigs fresh thyme

1 garlic clove, smashed

1. Preheat the oven to 400°F.

2. Pat the chicken breasts dry with paper towels, place between sheets of plastic wrap, and pound with a mallet for even cooking.

3. In a large cast-iron skillet, heat the grapeseed oil over medium-high heat. Season the chicken breasts with the salt and pepper. Add to the pan and cook until seared or caramelized on the outside, 5 to 6 minutes. Flip the chicken and add the butter, thyme, and garlic. Use a large spoon to baste the foaming butter over the chicken several times.

4. Transfer the chicken to the oven and roast until the internal temperature reaches 165°F, 12 to 15 minutes. Be sure to continue basting throughout the oven cooking time.

5. Allow the chicken to rest for 3 to 4 minutes before serving. Serve with a drizzle of butter from the pan.

Perfectly Pan-Roasted Proteins: Lamb Chops

This is one of my absolute favorite things to make for the family! When feeding a family, don't hesitate to ask the butcher to cut your lamb rack into chops. I love pairing lamb chops with quinoa pilaf (page 173). Or for a luxe touch, chill your serving bowls in the freezer before piling on a fresh, cool salad—the chilled bowls will keep it crisp—and topping it all with the hot lamb chops.

SERVES 2

4 lamb loin chops

2 tablespoons grapeseed oil

1 teaspoon sea salt

$1/2$ teaspoon ground black pepper

2 tablespoons grass-fed unsalted butter

4 sprigs fresh thyme

1 garlic clove, smashed

1. Remove the lamb chops from the fridge 20 to 30 minutes before cooking,

2. In a large skillet, heat the grapeseed oil over medium-high heat. Season the lamb chops with the salt and pepper. Cook the lamb chops undisturbed for 3 to 4 minutes on each side.

3. Add the butter, thyme, and garlic to the pan and cook, basting the lamb chops for 1 to 2 minutes. For medium-rare, remove the lamb chops from the heat and place on a plate to rest. Continue cooking for further doneness; medium-well will take 3 to 4 minutes longer.

Perfectly Pan-Roasted Proteins: Salmon

When grocery shopping for salmon, wild-caught is always the goal. Heather especially loves wild-caught Ora King salmon! To ensure juicy fish with crispy skin, score the skin of the fish using a very sharp knife. Serve and enjoy with a salad or cauliflower pilaf.

SERVES 2

1 tablespoon grapeseed oil

2 skin-on wild-caught salmon fillets (4 ounces each)

1 teaspoon sea salt

$1/2$ teaspoon ground black pepper

2 tablespoons grass-fed unsalted butter

4 sprigs fresh thyme

1 garlic clove, smashed

1. Preheat the oven to 400°F.

2. In a large ovenproof skillet, heat the grapeseed oil over medium-high heat. Season the salmon with the salt and pepper. Add the salmon to the pan skin-side down and cook undisturbed for 3 to 4 minutes. Add the butter, thyme, and garlic and cook, basting the fillets, for 1 minute.

3. Flip the salmon and transfer the pan to the oven and roast for 3 minutes for medium-rare, or continue cooking depending on your desired level of doneness. Be sure to baste once before removing the fish from the oven.

Avocado Butter

Butters and ghee can be stored in the refrigerator for up to 5 days and in the freezer for up to 6 months. I suggest cutting what you need for the week and storing the remainder of the log in the freezer. Make a couple of butters ahead and store them in the freezer for easy access.

This avocado butter is so delicious and pairs with the Pan-Roasted Salmon (page 185) and Pan-Roasted Chicken Breasts (page 183).

MAKES 8 OUNCES

1 avocado, halved and pitted

½ pound grass-fed unsalted butter, at room temperature

2 teaspoons minced shallots

1 tablespoon fresh lemon juice

2 teaspoons ground cumin

1 teaspoon sea salt

½ teaspoon ground black pepper

1. Scoop the avocado flesh into a bowl or food processor. Add the butter, shallots, lemon juice, cumin, salt, and pepper and mash everything together.

2. Transfer to a piece of parchment paper or plastic wrap. Roll the butter into a log and wrap it well. Twist the ends to secure. Refrigerate for at least 2 hours. Slice for serving.

Cajun Butter

Our Cajun Butter is a great addition to any of the Perfectly Pan-Roasted Proteins (pages 182–185). You can also add some to a pilaf for a zestier side dish.

MAKES 8 OUNCES

$1/2$ pound grass-fed unsalted butter, at room temperature

1 tablespoon chopped fresh parsley

2 teaspoons minced shallots

1 teaspoon chopped fresh thyme

1 tablespoon paprika

2 teaspoons garlic powder

1 teaspoon cayenne pepper

1 teaspoon brown sugar alternative

1 teaspoon sea salt

$1/2$ teaspoon ground black pepper

In a bowl (by hand) or with a food processor, combine all the ingredients well. Transfer to a piece of parchment paper or plastic wrap. Roll the butter into a log and wrap it well. Twist the ends to secure. Refrigerate for at least 2 hours. Slice for serving. Butter can be stored in the refrigerator for up to 5 days and in the freezer for up to 6 months.

Caramelized Onion & Herb Butter

This decadent butter is delicious with our Pan-Roasted Lamb Chops (page 184). Combine the two and enjoy with any of the grains for a fast and flavor-rich weeknight dinner.

MAKES 8 OUNCES

2 tablespoons olive oil

1 medium yellow onion, thinly sliced

1 1/2 teaspoons sea salt

1 teaspoon xylitol

1/2 pound grass-fed unsalted butter, at room temperature

1 tablespoon chopped fresh parsley

1/2 tablespoon chopped fresh thyme

1/2 teaspoon ground black pepper

1. In a nonstick skillet, heat the oil over medium-low to medium heat. Add the onion and sauté, stirring constantly, until beginning to brown and soften. Add 1/2 teaspoon of the salt and the xylitol and continue to cook until browned and sticky, 10 to 12 minutes. Remove from the heat and set aside to cool.

2. In a bowl (by hand) or in a food processor, combine the cooled caramelized onions, the butter, parsley, thyme, pepper, and remaining 1 teaspoon salt and combine well.

3. Transfer to a piece of parchment paper or plastic wrap. Roll the butter into a log and wrap it well. Twist the ends to secure. Refrigerate for at least 2 hours. Slice for serving. Butter can be stored in the refrigerator for up to 5 days and in the freezer for up to 6 months.

Anchovy & Herb Butter

Our Anchovy & Herb Butter is delicious when paired with one of our Perfectly Pan-Roasted Proteins (pages 182–185) and a fresh salad featuring romaine lettuce, arugula, or spinach. It's particularly great as a substitute for the butter in the chicken recipe (page 183).

MAKES 8 OUNCES

½ pound grass-fed unsalted butter, at room temperature

3 anchovy fillets, minced

2 teaspoons minced shallot

¾ tablespoon finely chopped fresh chives

¾ tablespoon finely chopped fresh parsley

2 teaspoons grated lemon zest

1 teaspoon red pepper flakes

1 teaspoon sea salt

½ teaspoon ground black pepper

In a bowl (by hand) or with a food processor, combine all the ingredients well. Transfer to a piece of parchment paper or plastic wrap. Roll the butter into a log and wrap it well. Twist the ends to secure. Refrigerate for at least 2 hours. Slice for serving. Butter can be stored in the refrigerator for up to 5 days and in the freezer for up to 6 months.

Olive & Herb Butter

This is definitely one of Heather's favorite compound butters with a crispy piece of Ora King salmon. It's also absolutely perfect as a substitute for plain butter in the recipes for Perfectly Pan-Roasted Proteins (pages 182–185), Grilled Chicken Thighs with Buttered Broccoli (page 169), and Spicy Mussels & Green Bean "Fries" (page 171).

MAKES 8 OUNCES

½ pound grass-fed unsalted butter, at room temperature

6 ounces Kalamata olives, chopped

¾ tablespoon chopped fresh rosemary

2 teaspoons grated lemon zest

1 teaspoon red pepper flakes

1 teaspoon sea salt

½ teaspoon ground black pepper

In a bowl (by hand) or with a food processor, combine all the ingredients well. Transfer to a piece of parchment paper or plastic wrap. Roll the butter into a log and wrap it well. Twist the ends to secure. Refrigerate for at least 2 hours. Slice for serving. Butter can be stored in the refrigerator for up to 5 days and in the freezer for up to 6 months.

Bacon, Parmesan & Herb Butter

This butter is especially delicious when substituted for plain butter in the Spicy Mussels & Green Bean "Fries" recipe (page 171). Try it— you will not be disappointed!

MAKES 8 OUNCES

$1/2$ pound grass-fed unsalted butter, at room temperature

2 slices uncured bacon, cooked and crumbled

$3/4$ tablespoon chopped fresh chives

2 tablespoons shaved parmesan cheese

1 teaspoon sea salt

$1/2$ teaspoon ground black pepper

In a bowl (by hand) or with a food processor, combine all the ingredients well. Transfer to a piece of parchment paper or plastic wrap. Roll the butter into a log and wrap it well. Twist the ends to secure. Refrigerate for at least 2 hours. Slice for serving. Butter can be stored in the refrigerator for up to 5 days and in the freezer for up to 6 months.

Hollandaise

This classic brunch sauce is truly delicious on our Pan-Roasted Rib Eyes (page 182), or when enjoyed with our Cauliflower Bacon Hash with Soft-Boiled Eggs (page 129).

MAKES 4 TO 5 OUNCES

2 large cage-free egg yolks

2 teaspoons fresh lemon juice

1/2 teaspoon mustard powder

1/4 pound grass-fed unsalted butter, melted and kept warm

1/2 teaspoon salt

1/2 teaspoon ground white pepper

In a blender, combine the yolks, lemon juice, mustard, and 1/2 tablespoon of water and mix well. With the machine running, slowly stream in the melted butter. Season with the salt and white pepper. Keep warm for serving. Leftover sauce can be stored in the refrigerator for up to 6 days.

Avocado & Basil Smash

Use this as a topping for our Pan-Roasted Salmon (page 185), and turn it into a great avocado toast spread by finishing it with chopped tomatoes. Kat loves making avocado toast for Coco and adding a fried egg on top!

MAKES 2½ CUPS

2 medium avocados, halved and pitted

½ cup fresh basil leaves

2 tablespoons fresh lime juice

1 teaspoon sea salt

½ teaspoon ground black pepper

Scoop the avocado flesh into a food processor, add the basil, lime juice, salt, and pepper and process to either chunky or smooth, depending on use. For avocado toast, for example, a chunky texture is best! Transfer to a glass storage dish and refrigerate or serve immediately. Leftovers can be stored in the refrigerator for up to 6 days.

Orange & Dill Infused Ghee

Kick up any of the grain pilafs by adding in some of this infused ghee. Everyone will be dying to know your secret ingredient!

MAKES 1 CUP

$^1/_2$ pound grass-fed unsalted butter

4 sprigs fresh dill

2 large strips orange zest

1. In a small saucepan, heat the butter over medium-low heat. When the butter begins to melt, add the dill and orange zest. When the butter has completely melted and white foamy solids begin rising to the top, skim off the foam with a long-handled spoon. Continue to cook the butter at a low simmer until it becomes golden and fragrant.

2. Line a fine-mesh sieve with cheesecloth and set over a bowl. Spoon the ghee into the sieve and discard the solids.

3. Allow the ghee to cool completely and store in an airtight glass container in the refrigerator for up to 5 days or in the freezer for up to 6 months.

CHAPTER 7

THE DKFD MEAL PLANS

To help you get a sense of how to combine meals and snacks to create the ideal day on the DKFD, we've provided three weeks' worth of meal plans. Try using the plans below to get yourself into a groove. Once you've tried a few varieties, you can make note of your favorite days so you can enjoy them again and again.

Of course, these meal plans aren't set in stone and you are encouraged to mix and match as long as you stick to the 8-hour Recharge recipes during the 8-hour window and 4-hour Refuel recipes during the 4-hour window. (I know this sounds so obvious, but just wanted to be sure it was clear!)

Week One

Day 1

Colla-Holla Latte (page 110)

Crispy Chicken Wings with Spicy Mustard Greens (page 139)

Bruschetta Topping & Herbed Cottage Cheese (page 157) served with Killer Kale Chips (page 117)

BBQ Shrimp with Walnut Broccolini (page 175)

Day 2

Morning Glory Coffee (page 111)

Fat Bomb Burger Sliders with Bacon-Wrapped Onion Rings (page 121)

Grilled Chicken Thighs with Buttered Broccoli (page 169)

Day 3

Coffee with 1 tablespoon cream

Bok Choy Salad with Pan-Seared Tofu (page 141)

Spicy Kale & Brazil Nut Dip (page 158) served with Golden Baked Zucchini Chips (page 116)

Spicy Mussels & Green Bean "Fries" (page 171)

Day 4

Coffee with 1 tablespoon cream

Parmesan & Dill Blinis with Smoked Salmon (page 126)

Billion Dollar Dip (page 160) served with Killer Kale Chips (page 117)

BBQ Shrimp with Walnut Broccolini (page 175)

Day 5

Colla-Holla Latte (page 110)

Southern-Style Shrimp & Cauliflower "Grits" (page 137)

White Turkey Chili over Cauliflower Cilantro "Rice" (page 167)

Herb & Tomato Salmon with Quinoa Pilaf (page 173)

Day 6

Iced Coffee (page 112)

Cauliflower Bacon Hash with Soft-Boiled Eggs (page 129)

Avocado Hummus (page 159) served with Crispy Okra Chips (page 115)

Beef & Kale Teriyaki with Cauliflower Fried "Rice" (page 161)

Day 7

Blended Iced Coffee with Coconut Whipped Cream (page 113)

Breakfast Salad with Ranch Dressing (page 123)

Grilled Flank Steak with Garden Vegetable Ratatouille (page 165)

Week Two

Day 1

Morning Glory Coffee (page 111)

Bacon & Parm Deviled Eggs (page 118) (2 servings = 6 egg halves)

Bacon & Roasted Garlic Kale Dip (page 156) served with Rosemary & Cracked Black Pepper Crackers (page 155)

Beef & Kale Teriyaki with Cauliflower Fried "Rice" (page 161)

Day 2

Coffee with 1 tablespoon cream

Parmesan & Dill Blinis with Smoked Salmon (page 126)

Avocado Hummus (page 159) served with Killer Kale Chips (page 117)

Pan-Roasted Lamb Chops (page 184) with Cajun Butter (page 187) and Garden Vegetable Ratatouille (page 165)

Day 3

Morning Glory Coffee (page 111)

Bacon-Wrapped Breakfast Burgers (page 127)

Grilled Chicken Thighs with Buttered Broccoli (page 169)

Day 4

Iced Coffee (page 112)

Breakfast Salad with Ranch Dressing (page 123)

Bacon & Roasted Garlic Kale Dip (page 156) served with Golden Baked Zucchini Chips (page 116)

Parmesan-Crusted Cod with "Invisible Rice" Pilaf (page 177)

Day 5

Colla-Holla Latte (page 110)

Cauliflower Bacon Hash with Soft-Boiled Eggs (page 129)

Zesty Coconut Lime Skirt Steak & Barley Fried "Rice" (page 163)

Day 6

Coffee with 1 tablespoon cream

Spinach Salad with Pan-Roasted Lamb Chops (page 133)

Loaded Celery Sticks (page 120)

Billion Dollar Dip (page 160) served with Rosemary & Cracked Black Pepper Crackers (page 155)

Pan-Roasted Salmon (page 185) with Spaghetti Squash with Parmesan & Pine Nuts (page 179)

Day 7

Coffee with 1 tablespoon cream

Cast-Iron Skillet Frittata (page 125)

Roasted Garlic Butter Steak Bites with Italian Mustard Greens (page 145)

Grilled Chicken Thighs with Buttered Broccoli (page 169)

My energy is the most valuable change I've seen so far—I can run circles around the woman I used to be!

—JESSI VALENTINO RELLO

Week Three

Day 1

Blended Iced Coffee with Coconut Whipped Cream (page 113)

Salmon & Avocado Poke with Green "Noodle" Salad (page 143)

Grilled Flank Steak with Garden Vegetable Ratatouille (page 165)

Day 2

Iced Coffee (page 112)

Southern-Style Shrimp & Cauliflower "Grits" (page 137)

Spicy Kale & Brazil Nut Dip (page 158) served with Killer Kale Chips (page 117)

White Turkey Chili over Cauliflower Cilantro "Rice" (page 167)

Day 3

Colla-Holla Latte (page 110)

Crispy Chicken Wings with Spicy Mustard Greens (page 139)

Bruschetta Topping & Herbed Cottage Cheese (page 157) served with Killer Kale Chips (page 117)

BBQ Shrimp with Walnut Broccolini (page 175)

Day 4

Coffee with 1 tablespoon cream

Cauliflower Bacon Hash with Soft-Boiled Eggs (page 129)

Spicy Kale & Brazil Nut Dip (page 158) served with Killer Kale Chips (page 117)

Pan-Roasted Chicken Breasts (page 183) served with Brown Rice Pilaf (page 181)

Day 5

Morning Glory Coffee (page 111)

Bacon-Wrapped Breakfast Burgers (page 127)

Grilled Chicken Thighs with Buttered Broccoli (page 169)

Day 6

Iced Coffee (page 112)

Fat Bomb Burger Sliders with Bacon-Wrapped Onion Rings (page 121)

Bruschetta Topping & Herbed Cottage Cheese (page 157) served with Killer Kale Chips (page 117)

Herb & Tomato Salmon with Quinoa Pilaf (page 173)

Day 7

Coffee with 1 tablespoon cream

Parmesan & Dill Blinis with Smoked Salmon (page 126)

Billion Dollar Dip (page 160) served with Killer Kale Chips (page 117)

BBQ Shrimp with Walnut Broccolini (page 175)

PART III

The DKFD Enhancers

CHAPTER 8

EXCLUSIVE WORKOUTS

In the first chapter, Terry mentioned the issue of too little—or minimal—exercise as one of the three primary factors contributing to the modern weight gain epidemic. As someone who used to be a non-exerciser, I would add that another consequence of minimal exercise is that you have limited energy and strength, and a general lack of stamina for whatever activities you may want to enjoy in your life. I was around forty-five when I started exercising regularly, and I've experienced so many incredibly profound improvements since then. These include a reduction in daily suffering from anxiety, increased strength and stamina, and an increase in happiness—I know that sounds silly, but it's true! I feel much better for knowing that I'm taking an active stance on improving my health every day, and it makes those indulgences—looking at you, brut champagne—all the more indulgent.

These benefits exist in addition to the ones that researchers have connected to exercise, like internal changes such as new nerve cells growing, reduced inflammation, improved metabolic function, healthier arteries, and improved mood and decreased effects of stress.

Since the DKFD introduces a diet that's higher in fat, which is naturally high in calories, it's recommended that you exercise regularly. A good general goal is to get in at least 30 minutes of exercise 5 days a week.

There are plenty of daily hacks for exercising more, such as opting to take the stairs instead of the elevator or taking a walk during your lunch break (or after dinner), but we're also big proponents of carving out space to exercise. And okay, we can be kind of intense about it.

Terry and I have talked a lot about how much we love high-intensity interval training (HIIT). This practice, which is based around periods of intense effort interspersed with short bursts of recovery, has become a favorite thanks to its efficiency and effectiveness. It's great for getting a quick, challenging, and head-clearing sweat session into your day.

But as Denny LeVine, Terry's personal trainer, shares below, high intensity isn't always the best to start out with when you're following even a keto-ish type of diet. You might eventually want to incorporate HIIT sessions, but it's best to start out with low- to moderate-intensity workouts as your metabolism adapts to a diet higher in fat and lower in carbs.

We asked Denny and my longtime personal trainer, Mona Arvanetis, to design exclusive workouts for the DKFD. These workouts are based on the very same ones they designed for Terry and me. Denny has provided a gym-based workout and Mona's will be suitable for at-home as it doesn't require gym equipment, but you might want to pick up some mini bands online to get the most out of the exercises she recommends.

Before we get to the workouts, I want to talk a little about the importance of investing in yourself as it relates to exercise, because I think this is an easy place to try to cut corners. You might justify so many other expenses before you say OK to spending money on workout classes or a personal trainer. But what other expense has the promise of being able to offer you easier weight control, disease prevention, better mood, more energy, improved sleep, increased interest in physical intimacy, and . . . FUN? My favorite thing I've found out about myself through exercise is that it keeps me from going totally crazy; seriously, exercise is my favorite way to manage—or reduce—stress.

Both Terry and I have been working with Denny and Mona off and on for several years. What I've found to be great about a trainer is that he or she can customize workouts to help you achieve a goal, whether it's to build strength, improve cardio health, or enhance flexibility . . . or a little of each of these. I'm not saying everyone has to have a trainer or needs to work out with one consistently, but I want to make a quick pitch for why you should consider one:

It's not as expensive as you think. A lot of people are under the impression that trainers are a luxury or cost a fortune, but that's not always the case. So many gyms have trainers on staff that you can hire for just a few sessions, or you can buy a bulk pack of sessions that will usually be cheaper than just one or two meetings.

It is the best way to learn form and prevent injury. You can find videos of so many exercises and workouts online, but this doesn't mean you can see a video of yourself trying them—and this is what matters. If your form isn't correct, you won't get as much out of a workout and, worse, you might get hurt.

It's like getting a workout and therapy at the same time. I've been going to my trainer Mona for over twelve years and she kicks my butt, but I also feel like I get a good soul workout as well. There are times when it's just you and your trainer, and for some reason you feel so free to be yourself. A trainer can be a good sounding board and push you to experience a purging from the inside out, and it's more than just a purging of sweat.

The bonus is that a trainer is often cheaper than a therapist—while it's not a substitute for therapy, personal training always delivers noticeable emotional as well as physical benefits.

You can find one that's right for you. If you're in the market for a trainer, seek out a couple of options and interview them. Ask their philosophy on bodies, and make sure they understand your goals and can help you achieve them. It's definitely worth investing in a great trainer, but do not spend money on someone who can't or won't help you get to your goals!

Try even just two sessions. As long as you can meet twice—once to get an initial evaluation and workout and then another time to run through the workout again and make sure your form is correct—I think it's worth it. More is better, but two workouts can establish a great foundation!

Find a good "app trainer." If you feel that hiring a trainer just isn't for you, there are so many fantastic apps now, too, that can provide workouts and quick video demonstrations on your phone. Check out Beachbody or FitPlan or search the app store for one with great reviews!

Go to a gym you like. This is more about the space in which you work out, but environment matters, too—if you're going to a gym for workouts, make it one you like. Do they play music you don't like? Does their lighting make you insane? Your exercise environment matters. If it's possible, shop around for a gym option that suits your taste. If it's not, get some good headphones and create your own headspace wherever it is you get to work out. As an added bonus, many gyms offer a free personal training session when you sign up.

Mona is one of the coolest chicks I know. She has a background in completive bodybuilding and genuinely loves helping people achieve their body goals. I've known Mona for over a decade, and she's been training me off and on in that time. She's seen me through my pregnancies and helped me recover my body after at least a couple of them. I always want her to target my glutes—I want a literal butt-kicking, or I should say lifting, workout just about every time—and Mona's always more than happy to give it to me. I'm super excited that she's contributing a workout for the DKFD!

Heather's Workout, by Mona Arvanetis

My name is Mona Arvanetis and I run Newport Workout out of Newport Beach, California, with my husband, Mike. We've been training people here for twenty-eight years! As Heather said, I come from the world of natural bodybuilding and I love helping people build health through strength. Like I always tell Heather, "a strong body is a young body." When I design workouts for her, I'm helping her improve endurance, flexibility, energy, and strength and also helping her prevent injury. We achieve this with bands, weights, planking, and bodyweight workouts.

For this book, I'm sharing one of the bodyweight workouts I've created for her, which will help you strengthen and build your core and lower body (hips, inner and outer thighs, and butt). This workout has just eight exercises, which means you can do one round quickly or more rounds if you have additional time. One round should take you about 30 minutes. You can do this three times a week.

Since there's no need for any gym equipment, the workout can be done at home or in the stretching/sit-up space at your gym. I have included mini bands because they are so fantastic for creating resistance, but you can get started without these. You can find mini bands online or at a local sporting goods store.

You are going to start the workout by doing each of these 3 poses for 30 seconds, and then repeating (total of 2 minutes):

Downward-Facing Dog

Get on your hands and knees (use a mat if you're on a hard surface), aligning your hands directly under your shoulders and knees directly under your hips. Exhale as you tuck your toes and lift your knees off the floor, reaching your pelvis up toward the ceiling. Push your sit bones (the bones at the base of your butt) back and up to bring your body into the shape of an A. Keep your hands shoulder-distance apart; feet hip-distance apart. Activate your upper arms by externally rotating them. Keep your neck and head along the same line as the spine, shoulder blades firm, and upper back wide. Engage the lower belly by drawing the navel in toward the spine. Bend knees a little (or a lot) and send the sit bones and tailbone up and back.

Plank Pose

This is an arm-balancing yoga pose that tones the abdominal muscles while strengthening the arms and spine. Plank pose engages all of the core muscles of the body. Get into a push-up position; arms should be shoulder-distance apart, your feet hip-distance apart. You can hold the pose with your palms flat on the ground or lower to your forearms.

Upward-Facing Dog

Lie facedown, legs and feet fully extended. With your elbows and palms pressed into the ground, inhale as you straighten your arms, lifting your torso. Legs should also be lifted a few inches off the floor.

With these next five exercises, you'll work on creating a little burn in your muscles.

Three-Legged Downward Dog Kickback

Complete 1 to 3 sets of 10 to 20 reps.
Add a mini band for an extra challenge.

Get on your hands and knees, aligning your hands directly under your shoulders and knees directly under your hips. Exhale as you tuck your toes and lift your knees off the floor, reaching your pelvis up toward the ceiling. Draw your hips back to bring your body into the shape of an A. Keep your standing leg strong and shoulders squared to the floor. Lift your other leg up toward the sky with a 5-pound ankle weight (or no weight). Kick toward your butt and then up toward the sky. Repeat on the other leg.

Lateral Walk

Complete 3 sets of 20 reps.

Place a mini band around your ankles so it is lying flat against the legs. Stand with your feet about shoulder width apart so the mini band gets a little tension in it. Bend your knees slightly, keeping your hips back and your head and chest up.

Take a large step out to the left, keeping your feet in line with your shoulders, your hips level, and your weight evenly distributed. This large step will cause a good amount of tension in the mini band. Follow that large step with a smaller step to the left with your opposite foot, closing the gap slightly without losing tension.

Continue doing these steps to the left for 20 reps. And then complete to the right for 20 reps. This will be one set.

If you don't have a mini band, simply practice the lateral walk without it, but be sure to focus on maintaining a slight bend in your knees.

Lateral Leg Raise

Complete 1 to 3 sets of 10 to 20 reps.

Slide the mini band over both feet and up around the ankles so it is flat against the legs. Lie on the ground, positioning yourself on your right side with both legs straight, your left leg directly on top of your right. You can put your right arm behind your head and your left arm on the floor in front of you for support.

Raise your left leg as high as you can without moving any other part of your body. Once you get tension in the band and your leg is as high as it can go without breaking form, return your left leg to the starting position in a controlled manner. Repeat on the other side.

Squat

Complete 3 sets of 20 reps.

Slide a mini band around both feet and pull the band up just above your knees. Stand with your feet shoulder width apart and keep your head and chest up (no hunching over).

Sit your hips back, bending at your knees. Push your knees out and against the mini band as you squat and try to get your thighs parallel to the ground. Once you get parallel, push through your hips and return to the starting position.

Glute Bridge

Complete 3 sets of 20 reps.

Put a mini band around both feet and pull the band up just above your knees. Lie on the floor face up with your knees bent to 90 degrees, feet flat on the floor and arms out to your sides. Spread your legs apart slightly so there is tension in the mini band.

Raise your hips off the ground until your knees, hips, and shoulders are all in a straight line; pause at the top of the lift and then slowly lower yourself back down to the starting position. Keep tension in the mini band throughout the entire exercise.

> *Denny LeVine is the man. He's been training me now for about seven years, and came as a recommendation when my earlier trainer was moving out of state. Denny knows what I like—high-intensity circuit training. And he doesn't take it easy on me, not even for a second. I'll let him tell you a little more about himself and the workouts he's designed for the DKFD.*

Dr. Dubrow's Workout, by Denny LeVine

My name is Denny LeVine. I am a certified personal trainer with a bachelor of science degree in kinesiology, exercise science, from California State University, Long Beach. I have been working with Dr. Dubrow for seven years. His favorite type of workout is high-intensity circuit training, and his goal in the gym is to maintain a fit, athletic physique without getting too bulky.

The workouts we're including in this book are designed to produce the same outcome. If your body goal is to create an athletic, lean, well-balanced physique, these are ideal for you. But again— they're not about becoming bulky; we are aiming for "fit" and trying to stay as youthful as possible. Remember, in a lot of ways youth isn't about age, but ability.

Dr. Dubrow also needs workouts that are as efficient as possible and allow him to maximize his time in the gym, and the workouts here will help you do the same.

To make sure that your exercising supports how you are eating on the Dubrow Keto Fusion Diet, you will want to pay attention to your intensity level, which you can gauge based on how hard you are breathing, how much you are sweating, and how fatigued your muscles feel. Intensity plays a huge role in determining which macronutrient is utilized as fuel. While Dr. Dubrow performs these workouts at a high intensity, he's been training hard for a long time and likely has a metabolic flexibility that allows him to stay in fat-burning mode most of the time.

If you are an untrained individual, I recommend starting at a lower intensity and working up to the higher intensity intervals, which will allow the body to get conditioned for the workouts. This is important because we want the body using fat for fuel, and if the workouts are too intense for one's current level of fitness, it will be burning mostly glycogen (stored glucose from carbs) instead. This specific combination of diet and exercise is designed to turn the body into a fat-burning machine.

The workouts are structured so that each day is a full-body workout that involves both anaerobic and aerobic training, and generally take about 45 minutes. You'll use standard gym equipment including free weights, machines, cable pulleys, and exercise balls.

DR. DUBROW'S WORKOUT A: PUSH

3 rounds per circuit before moving to next circuit (circuits are separated by black lines). 10 to 15 reps per set; 20 reps for abs. No rest between exercises; 60-second rest between circuits.

Machine Fly	Dumbbell Chest Press
Machine Chest Press	Hack Squat
Dumbbell Goblet Squat	Cable Chest Fly
Incline Dumbbell Press	Push-Up
Leg Press	Cable Wood Chop
Cable Triceps Push-Down	Ab Crunch Machine
Standing Military Press	Decline Reverse Crunch

DR. DUBROW'S WORKOUT B: PULL

3 rounds per circuit before moving to next circuit. 10 to 15 reps per set; 20 reps for abs. No rest between exercises; 60-second rest between circuits.

V-Bar Cable Pull-Down	Standing Biceps Cable Curl
Deadlift	Single-Arm Dumbbell Row
Reverse Machine Fly	Lying Leg Curl
Machine Row	Lower Back Extension
Dumbbell Lateral Raise	Hanging Pike
Leg Press	Exercise Ball Rolling Plank
Incline Dumbbell Row	Exercise Ball Crunch
Rope Straight-Arm Pull-Down	

Machine Fly

1. Choose your weight and adjust the seat so that your hands are right about where your chest and abs meet. Make sure the handles are back far enough to fully stretch your chest.

2. Grab the handles, keeping your elbows and arms parallel to the floor. Roll your shoulders back and down as much as possible while keeping your chest up and back against the seat.

3. Exhale as you bring your hands together in a hugging motion. Be sure to squeeze and contract your chest as much as possible at the top of the motion.

4. Return back to the starting position as you control the weight down, keeping tension on the muscle the entire time. Do not let the weight stack touch at the bottom.

5. Repeat the exercise until the recommended number of sets and reps are completed.

Machine Chest Press

1. Adjust the machine so the hands are at mid-chest level before adding the weight. Once adjusted, select your desired weight.

2. Start by pressing your shoulders back and down as you raise your chest. Your elbows should be close to your body.

3. Lift the weight by contracting the chest, imagining trying to touch the biceps together.

4. Squeeze and contract the chest at the top without locking the elbows, then lower the weight down, slow and controlled, keeping tension on the muscles.

5. Repeat the exercise until the recommended number of sets and reps are completed.

Dumbbell Goblet Squat

1. Start by standing with your feet slightly wider than shoulder width apart. With both hands, cradle the head of a dumbbell close to your chest. Your back should be straight with your head up and shoulders pulled slightly back.

2. Squat as if you were sitting in a chair, making sure to keep your head and chest up and shoulders back. Lower until your butt is in line with your knees.

3. Exhale and press from the heels as you squeeze your glutes and hamstrings to return to the top without locking out, as this will keep the tension in the muscle.

4. Repeat the exercise until the recommended number of sets and reps are completed.

Incline Dumbbell Press

1. Set the bench to about a 30-degree angle. With a dumbbell in each hand, lie back using your knees to kick the dumbbells up one at a time to your shoulders. Your palms should be facing slightly forward.

2. Press your shoulders back and down as you raise your chest; keep your elbows close to your body.

3. Exhale as you contract your chest to press the weights up and together at the top, keeping the elbows from flaring out. Do not lock out at the top.

4. Control the weights back down to the starting position, maintaining constant tension on the chest.

5. After the number of reps have been completed, lower the dumbbells down to the shoulders and bring the knees up at the same time to allow the momentum to propel you up to where you started.

6. Repeat the exercise until the recommended number of sets are completed.

Leg Press

1. On the leg press machine, adjust the back support to the desired angle then load the desired weight. Sit on the machine with your back firmly pressed into the seat. Place your feet on the platform, one foot at a time, about shoulder width apart. Pressing from the heels, drive the weight up from the resting position and unlock the safety levers.

2. Inhale as you lower the weight in a controlled manner, pausing for 2 seconds at the bottom.

3. Exhale as you press the weight back up, driving from the heels, making sure not to lock out at the top. Tip: Slightly lift the toes to keep the heels focused on driving the weight.

4. Repeat the exercise until the recommended number of sets and reps are completed.

Cable Triceps Push-Down

1. Set the pulley to the highest position and attach a straight or angled bar. Grab the bar with your hands down-grip and elbows in tight, head and chest up.

2. Exhale and squeeze the triceps to press the bar down, keeping the chest up and making sure the elbows don't drift.

3. Squeeze and contract the triceps as much as possible at bottom of the movement.

4. Repeat the exercise until the recommended number of sets and reps are completed.

Standing Military Press

1. Adjust the barbell so that it racks just at shoulder level then load the desired weight. Grip the barbell with the hands about shoulder width apart, palms facing forward.

2. Unrack the barbell by stepping under it slightly. Lift the bar to your collarbone and take a small step back, posi-

tioning your feet shoulder width apart, elbows slightly forward.

3. Keep your back straight and abs tight and exhale as you press the bar up overhead. Do not fully lock out.

4. Control the weight down to chin level keeping the tension on the deltoids (the muscles that form the front part of your shoulder).

5. Repeat the exercise until the recommended number of sets and reps are completed.

Dumbbell Chest Press

1. On a flat bench, grasp a dumbbell in each hand. Lie back using your knees to kick the dumbbells up, one at a time, to your shoulders with your palms facing slightly forward.

2. Press your shoulders back and down as you raise your chest. Your elbows should be close to your body.

3. Exhale as contract your chest to press the weights up and together at the top, keeping the elbows from flaring out. Do not lock out at the top.

4. Control the weights back down to the starting position, keeping constant tension on the chest.

5. Repeat the exercise until the recommended number of sets and reps are completed.

Hack Squat

1. Load the weight onto a hack squat machine and then step into the machine, getting in position with your knees slightly bent. Walk your feet slightly forward with feet shoulder width apart, shoulders and back comfortably against the pads.

2. Release the safety levers and unrack the weight but do not lock the knees out.

3. Inhale as you bend your knees squatting down through a full range of motion at the bottom until your butt is in line with your knees.

4. Exhale and press from the heels as you squeeze your glutes, hamstrings, and quads to return to the top without locking out so that the tension stays on the muscle. Tip: Focus on keeping the lower back pressed against the pads to keep stress off the spine and avoid having the knee drift over the toes to keep the stress off the knees.

5. Repeat the exercise until the recommended number of sets and reps are completed.

Cable Chest Fly

1. Set the cables to their highest position and attach the handle grips to each side. Pick the desired weight (use a lighter weight on this exercise). Stand in the middle with the handles in each hand.

2. With a slight bend at the waist, step forward one step then pull the handles together into your chest and extend out with palms facing forward. From here, lower the weight in an arc motion, creating a full stretch in the chest.

3. Exhale as you bring your hands together in front in a hugging motion, keeping a slight bend in the elbows. Squeeze and contract the chest at the peak of the motion.

4. Repeat the exercise until the recommended number of sets and reps are completed.

Push-Up

1. Lie on the floor facedown and place your hands palms down about shoulder width apart. With your abs tight and back straight, press yourself up into a push-up position.

2. Keeping tension on your chest, lower yourself down until your chest is just about to touch the ground.

3. Exhale as you press the ground away by contracting your chest and try to visualize touching your biceps together.

4. Repeat the exercise until the recommended number of sets and reps are completed.

Cable Wood Chop

1. On a cable machine, attach a handle to the pulley and set it to the highest level.

2. With one shoulder pointing toward the pulley, grab the handle with the hand farthest away first then cradle the other hand around and extend the arms out. Take one step away from the pulley to create tension with your feet slightly wider than shoulder width.

3. Exhale as you rotate the torso in a downward twisting motion, initiating the rotation by using the obliques to drive the movement.

4. Keeping the resistance on the obliques and the arms extended, return back to the starting position without letting the weight rack touch.

5. Repeat the exercise until the recommended number of reps are completed, then perform the same amount of reps on the other side to complete one set.

Ab Crunch Machine

1. Sit down on the machine and adjust it to the desired height, then select a light to medium weight.

2. Exhale and crunch, bringing the elbows and knees together by contracting the abs, and hold and squeeze at the peak of the motion. Tip: Visualize your abs flexing to drive

the movement to minimize the lower back coming into the exercise.

3. Return back to the starting position in a controlled manner.

4. Repeat the exercise until the recommended number of reps and sets are completed.

Decline Reverse Crunch

1. Start by lying on a decline bench, gripping the sides of the bench. Hold yourself in this position with a slight bend in the knees.

2. Exhale as you drive your knees up toward your elbows using your lower abdominals.

3. Squeeze and contract at the peak of the movement when your knees are touching your elbows.

4. Lower your legs back to the starting position without letting your feet touch the ground.

5. Repeat the exercise until the recommended number of sets and reps are completed.

V-Bar Cable Pull-Down

1. Attach a V-bar to a lat pull-down machine. Grip the handles with the palms, focusing the grip on your three outside fingers and allowing the index fingers and thumbs to relax into a kind of pistol grip. Sit into the knee supports.

2. With your arms fully extended, let the lats (the big flat muscles that attach to your mid spine on your back and extend to your sides) relax and stretch completely.

3. Exhale as you retract your shoulder blades down and together, pulling from the elbows and lats. Allow your chest to extend up as you pull the bar down to the top of your

collarbone. It's very important to squeeze at the peak of the contraction for a full second count.

4. Resist the weight while lowering it back to the starting position, allowing the resistance to pull and stretch the lats completely.

5. Repeat the exercise until the recommended number of sets and reps are completed.

Deadlift

1. Load the weight onto a barbell. You'll want to begin with a light weight to warm up then progress the weight with each set. With your hands shoulder width apart grip the bar with one hand over and the other hand under (alternate this hand position on each set). Your feet should also be about shoulder width apart.

2. Bend your knees and lift your head and chest. It's important to keep the head and chest up throughout the entire exercise. Engage the core and exhale as you drive the bar up by imagining pushing the ground away from your heels, keeping the bar close against the body. Squeeze the glutes and lower back at the top of the motion.

3. Keeping the head and chest up, lower the bar back to the ground in a controlled manner then explode into the next rep.

4. Repeat the exercise until the recommended number of sets and reps are completed.

Reverse Machine Fly

1. Set the handles to their farthest back position. Sit with your face toward the pad, and then grab the handles and extend

them out with the palms facing inward. Be sure the seat is low enough so that the hands are at the same level as the shoulders.

2. Drive the handles back by contracting the rear delts keeping the elbows from dipping and maintaining constant tension on the rear delts. Squeeze and contract at the peak of the motion.

3. Lower the weight back to the starting position, not letting the weight stack touch.

4. Repeat the exercise until the recommended number of sets and reps are completed.

Machine Row

1. Select the desired weight and adjust the seat height so that the handles are at chest level. Grip the handles, allowing the index fingers and thumbs to relax into a kind of pistol grip.

2. With your arms fully extended, let the lats relax and stretch completely. Exhale as you retract your shoulders down and together, pulling from the elbows and lats. Allow your chest to extend up as you pull the bar into your torso. It's very important to squeeze at the peak of the contraction for a full second count.

3. Resist the weight while lowering it back to the starting position, allowing the resistance to pull and stretch the lats completely.

4. Repeat the exercise until the recommended number of sets and reps are completed.

Dumbbell Lateral Raise

1. Stand with a dumbbell in each hand, palms facing back.

2. Keeping a slight bend in the elbows, raise the weights up

and out to the sides at shoulder level but not higher. Never let the dumbbell go higher than the elbow. Tip: Turn the thumbs down as you raise the weight as if you were pouring out a cup of water.

3. Lower the dumbbells, slow and controlled, back down to the starting position, never taking the tension off the delts.

4. Repeat the exercise until the recommended number of sets and reps are completed.

Incline Dumbbell Row

1. Set the incline bench to about a 30-degree angle with a dumbbell on each side.

2. Lie facedown on the bench and grab the dumbbells in each hand with the palms facing each other.

3. With your arms fully extended let the lats relax and stretch completely. Exhale as you retract your shoulders back and together, pulling from the elbows and lats as if you were trying to put a coin in your front pocket. It's very important to squeeze at the peak of the contraction for a full second count.

4. Repeat the exercise until the recommended number of sets and reps are completed.

Rope Straight-Arm Pull-Down

1. Select the desired weight and set the pulley to the highest setting with a rope attached. Take one side of the rope in each hand and take a few steps back to fully stretch the lats. Bend at the waist just a little.

2. Exhale and drive the rope down toward your thighs, keeping your arms straight and pulling with the lats. It's very important to squeeze at the peak of the contraction for a full second count.

3. Return to the starting position without allowing the weight to fully rest on the stack.

4. Repeat the exercise until the recommended number of sets and reps are completed.

Standing Biceps Cable Curl

1. Set the pulley to the lowest level with a curl bar attached. Grab the bar with the palms up, standing with a slight foreword bend at the waist and elbows firmly by the sides.

2. Curl the bar up by contracting the biceps (the only part of the arm that should move is from the elbow to the fingertip). Keep the elbows from drifting as well. Squeeze and contract the biceps as hard as possible at the peak.

3. Lower the weight back to the starting position, never taking tension off the biceps.

4. Repeat the exercise until the recommended number of sets and reps are completed.

Single-Arm Dumbbell Row

1. Select a desired dumbbell and set it near a flat bench. Place one knee on the bench and lean forward with one arm extended on the bench, keeping your head and chest up.

2. Grab the dumbbell with the other hand and row the weight up and back as if you were trying to put a coin in your front pocket. It's very important to squeeze at the peak of the contraction for a full second count.

3. Lower the weight back down to the starting position in a controlled manner, fully stretching the lats.

4. Repeat the exercise until the recommended number of reps are completed, then perform the same amount of reps on the other side to complete one set.

Lying Leg Curl

1. Lie facedown on the leg curl machine and adjust the pad so it's just between your calf and ankle and grab the handles.
2. Exhale as you curl the weight up by contracting with your hamstrings. Squeeze and contract at the top of the movement.
3. Return the weight back to the starting position, keeping the tension on the hamstrings and never allowing the weights to touch the rack.
4. Repeat the exercise until the recommended number of sets and reps are completed.

Lower Back Extension

1. Adjust a hyperextension bench so that the pad is just below hip level.
2. Cross your arms and bend at the waist keeping your head and chest up.
3. Lift your torso up by squeezing and contracting the lower back and hold the contraction at the top of the movement. Tip: For more resistance, extend the arms out in front or hold a weight to your chest.
4. Repeat the exercise until the recommended number of sets and reps are completed.

Hanging Pike

1. Hang from a pull-up bar with a slight bend in your knees.
2. Engage the abs and exhale as you draw your legs up toward the bar as high as possible.
3. Return back to the starting position in a controlled manner trying to keep your body from swinging.
4. Repeat the exercise until the recommended number of sets and reps are completed.

Exercise Ball Rolling Plank

1. Place your elbows onto an exercise ball and extend your body until you are in a plank position so that the elbows are directly under the shoulders.
2. Engage the abs and exhale as you push the ball out and away from your body (about 6 inches). Squeeze and hold here at the peak of the movement then draw the elbows back to the starting position.
3. Repeat the exercise until the recommended number of sets and reps are completed.

Exercise Ball Crunch

1. Sit upright on an exercise ball then walk your feet forward and roll your body down the ball until you feel support in your lower back. Lift the chin and head just a bit and cross your arms in front of you.
2. Lower your torso and fully stretch the abs keeping your head and chin up.
3. Engage the abs and exhale as you crunch up toward the ceiling. Squeeze and hold here at the peak of the movement.
4. Return back to the starting position in a controlled manner, keeping tension on the abs throughout the entire exercise.
5. Repeat the exercise until the recommended number of sets and reps are completed.

I'm starting to feel like me again—my clothes are fitting better and people are noticing. I'm feeling so much more confident.

—SHARON GROSSWIRTH COPPOLA

HOW TO SUPPORT YOUR SUCCESS FROM THE INSIDE OUT

When you want to create sustainable success in any area of your life, you have to prioritize the foundation first. For example, if you want a good job, you have to build a foundation of education and skill; if you want a great relationship, you have to first stabilize your sense of self. The same is true with any type of health-related goal, whether it's weight loss or something else: You've got to lay the groundwork for success; it doesn't just happen without that in place.

In our own lives, Terry and I have learned to create a solid foundation for success by doing the internal work that will help get the external results we want. We support our internal health in two ways: (1) by taking care of our emotional well-being (because if you don't feel right in the head, it's so much harder to take action for your health) and (2) by taking care of our internal cellular health with selective supplements that can cover all the gaps left behind by even a nutrient-rich diet.

Here are some of the specific ways we establish a foundation strong enough to support the kind of active, vibrant, fulfilling, and fun-filled lives we want to lead.

How to Take Care of Your Internal Emotional Health

Everyone's got their own bag of tricks to help them make it through this crazy thing called life. And sometimes we have to reach extra deep into that bag to find what we need, not just to keep going but also to keep pursuing our best selves.

Some people find what they need in God and religion; this is what helps them manage their day-to-day existence and get through all things big and small and gives them that extra oomph to start something new and stick with it.

Other people lean more on self-help practices, like meditation and therapy, to stay grounded and motivated. Still other people find it most helpful, when they have a problem or question, to turn to their family or friends, or to reach outside of their immediate circle and connect online or in person with others who are going through the same experience. This "experience" could be anything, whether it's a quest for parenting advice, workout inspiration, or dieting support. I know people love connecting on our Facebook page for this program and sharing and discussing tips or special tricks.

What works really varies from person to person. What's important is that you find something that works for *you*.

Sometimes what's worked for you before stops working, and that's scary! That's what happened to me over the last couple of years, thanks to waking up and suddenly being in my late forties . . . *how did that happen?* The hormonal turmoil of this time had left me emotionally and physically out of whack. In a way, it's similar to any big life change—there's an imbalance, followed by a transition, followed by an adjustment period. The question remains the same no matter what that big change is: How do you ground yourself?

I know it might sound crazy, but you know what I found that works for me? Going to a psychic medium. I know, I know, this is something I *never* thought I would be into. But I started going to this woman, Mrs. Lee, just on a whim. For whatever reason, I felt open to whatever this woman might introduce into my life. I believe and don't believe in it at the same time . . . but if you believe in something, I think you can make it true.

Going to her became the kind of therapy I needed at the time. She created a space where I could talk about my deepest fears and greatest desires, and she gave me the tools to use when I needed them. She helped me regain a little bit of stability in the middle of some rocky seas, and that stability was what let me get back into taking better care of myself and my family. Again, this isn't an actual suggestion to go to a tarot card reader—but it is a reminder to keep an open mind about where you might find support when you need it. Take my psychic experience as an example—you just can't know what will work for you until you get outside of your comfort zone!

If you are in a place where you feel like you need to fortify your emotional well-being so you can take care of your physical health, there are so many ways to go about this. You can:

Take advantage of the dozens of amazing inspirational people out there sharing their message. There are so many podcasts and books these days that are full of positive methods of self-betterment; don't be afraid to dig into any of these to help boost your emotional well-being. Even if you have people in your life who are supportive, sometimes you just need to hear it from someone else. It's like when your mom would tell you, "You're special," and you'd say, "You have to say that, you're my mom"—you don't really hear it from someone close to you because you doubt the sincerity or truth of the message. Sometimes you need a stranger to tell you with confidence—you're worthy and you can do this; you can bring your potential to life.

Try meditation (or anything that induces a meditative state). I know a lot of people use meditation, specifically transcendental meditation, to help them stay grounded and sane, and this might be something that works for you. I've never been able to get into it, but Terry has practiced it for a long time and he finds it extraordinarily helpful (of course, he tells me he does it in his own "Terry-ish" way, whatever that means!). What I have found works for me to create a meditative state is singing; when I'm singing is really the only time I can't think about anything else. Other people talk about how knitting or coloring in adult coloring books can create a sort of Zen state. Seek and find your thing.

Define your goal, in words and pictures. Establishing your goal is another way to strengthen your internal sense of purpose. If you've ever taken a yoga class, you know that teachers often tell you to pick a point out in front of you to stare at during a balancing pose, and this point of focus will help you hold the pose. I think having a goal works much the same way—it just gives you a stabilizing point of reference.

As you begin the DKFD, do you know what your goal is? I know I mentioned that we really try to stay on top of our game healthwise because we want to be around for our kids. But I also have another goal and that is to look as hot as I can for as long as I can, and I don't have any shame in saying this! There's nothing wrong with the vanity of wanting to look good, because looking good makes you feel good.

Maybe your goal is about health or looks or a mashup of the

two, which is perfect because the two often go hand in hand. Who knows? Next time you have a free moment, take a seat at the kitchen table and write down some of the things you want from life. These could be for the short or long term, whatever comes to mind. Once you've finished writing the list, put it in a drawer. Wait a couple of days, take out the piece of paper, and choose the items that your now-refreshed self sees as the most important components of your goal.

Once you define your goal, get a whiteboard or at least a journal and write it down. Take your "before" picture and tack it on your whiteboard or staple it into your journal and get set up to track your diet progress. You can add lines to jot down your weight once a week or a space where you can write a few words about how you feel, whether you're having challenges or wins, big or small.

One other idea that you can have a lot of fun with is creating a Pinterest board and filling it with ideas of how you want to look and feel. Scroll for some images of people around your age who inspire you—whether with their strength or their style or just the overall statement they make—and save these. Or you can go old school and cut out pictures from magazines and paste them in a journal. Some people might tell you to find a picture of how you used to look and aim for that, but I think that's a slippery slope . . . and not one that slopes in a positive direction. I like to say, what if the best version of you is still to come?

Become a preparation ninja. While telling you to be prepared doesn't exactly sound like advice that relates to emotional well-being, it is probably one of the most powerful ways to prevent panic around falling off track.

When you're getting prepped to start the DKFD, you'll need to carve out time for food prep and time to go to the grocery store and so on. Beyond that, I encourage you to be prepared with your schedule as well by always looking to what's coming up each week and planning ahead. I laminated a calendar so I could write on it each week with all the kids' schedules and our plans as a couple. I hung it in our pantry and this way I can take a look at events, lunches, dinners, etc. that are coming up and prepare for them. I can scan and see where my challenges may be.

When you're first trying to stick to a specific eating plan, it seems like challenges lurk around every single corner. Let's say your sister-in-law picked a restaurant for dinner next week that you think will never work for your diet . . . what do you do? First, you pull up the menu online and you see what you can order—there's always something that will work: Grilled steak, fish, or chicken and some veggies cooked in butter or oil are consistent safe bets. You can even call the restaurant in advance and ask if you can make modifications; that way you don't feel embarrassed in the moment and make a bad choice. Like I said—become a preparation ninja. Things don't have to be difficult or derail your progress if you plan ahead.

So, those are some of the ways to support your internal emotional health as you get started on this plan. You might also want to think about incorporating some supplements to support your internal cellular health. Both can be helpful in creating remarkable external results.

How We Support Our Diet with Supplements

I used to be a little meh on supplements. I thought they couldn't possibly be helpful enough to justify the need to create a daily habit of pill-popping (granted, I used to have a habit of drinking Diet Cokes and smoking cigarettes . . . but you know, it's funny how we decide what we want to define as a difficult habit to stick with). Then I got a little older and I started to feel the effects of aging. It wasn't that I felt old and incapable or anything dramatic like that . . . it's just that I started to feel a little less stellar than my normal self. So I started to explore what types of supplements I could take that would maybe help the health of my skin, hair, and nails, and maybe boost my energy levels. Then, of course, as the years kept climbing, I started thinking about needing something for my joints and then something to address the loss of natural suppleness in my face . . . ugh, the list just keeps getting longer! But that's OK—working to outsmart the effects of aging beats not aging all day long. Right?

Your priorities as you approach your health should be: Follow a good diet (the one in this book works!), drink a lot of water every day, exercise so that you break a sweat almost every day, and then, if your physician gives the go-ahead, add in some supplements to help support your internal cellular health and fill in any gaps in your diet.

We're including here some of our favorite supplements that we take daily. Some of these are old standbys that you've probably heard a lot about, but others are newer ones that we've recently grown to like. Since people often ask what we personally take, we'll include info about those, which are from our own brand called Consult Beaute. But you can absolutely find and take whatever brand you want to try!

And with that, I'm going to let Terry jump in here to share with you some brief but detailed info about the supplements we take each day.

Multivitamin. When I'm in surgery all day, it's almost impossible for me to get enough nutrition-rich food into my body to support all the metabolic functions taking place there. Usually I'm fasting a good chunk of the time, and my cells seem to have adjusted to doing without food for hours on end. But they still have nutrient needs, which I try to meet with supplements such as a multivitamin. I look for a multivitamin that's going to provide vitamins A, C, D, E, B_6, B_{12}, thiamin, riboflavin, and folic acid; the minerals zinc, magnesium, iron, selenium, chromium, copper, sodium, and potassium; and MSM (or at least a lot of this good stuff!).

Vitamin D_3. Deficiency in vitamin D has been linked to anxiety and depression, decreased bone mass, and some types of cancer, and may contribute to increased risk of developing type 2 diabetes. If you are dark skinned or obese or spend a lot of time indoors (i.e., you don't get 15 minutes of daily sunscreen-free sun exposure, which you need to facilitate production of vitamin D), you are more likely to develop a deficiency.

The only way to know if you are currently deficient is to have your levels checked by a blood test administered at your doctor's office (this is a level worth the attention). And if you are going to start supplemental vitamin D_3, I highly recommend testing where you stand beforehand. This way, you can establish a starting point and see what kind of improvements are made by a daily dose. I generally suggest a dose of 3,000 to 5,000 IU, but ask your doctor for a specific recommendation based on your current levels.

Coenzyme Q10. Coenzyme Q10, or CoQ10 as it's also known, is a compound that's naturally present in every cell and tissue found in the body. As a "co"-enzyme, it helps an enzyme do its job. In this way, it is essential to energy production and the protection of cell membranes and DNA.

In research, CoQ10 supplementation has been shown to help improve blood vessel health, which could translate to lowered risk of heart disease. It has also been found to lower blood pressure, reduce the side effects of statins, and decrease the risk of a second heart attack. All this is to say, I think it's a really good supplement. As with vitamin D, you can get your levels checked by your doctor to determine if supplementation will benefit you. I generally suggest a daily dose of 200 mg of CoQ10. Be sure to get a brand that also contains piperine, sometimes listed as Bioperine on the label, which is a pepper plant extract that can increase absorption of CoQ10.

Biotin. This water-soluble B vitamin is important to hair, skin, and nail health, and is essential to the metabolism of macronutrients, which is how you get the energy your body needs to function. If you don't have enough available biotin, you may experience brittle nails and hair loss, and you could be at increased risk of developing type 2 diabetes. Many pregnant and breastfeeding women will develop a borderline biotin deficiency due to greater demands for this vitamin during pregnancy. Heather certainly experienced a biotin deficiency after pregnancy and relied heavily on biotin supplementation to help restore her hair and nail health.

We like to take a biotin supplement that offers around 8,000 mcg (micrograms). If you have type 2 diabetes, you could consider trying one that's combined with chromium picolinate as biotin plus chromium may improve blood sugar levels (we love chromium and used it in our Carb-ology product; see more about this on page 45).

Collagen. Collagen is one of those things about which you can say, "You don't know what you have until it's gone." As one of the most abundant proteins in your body, collagen is responsible for skin elasticity and provides essential cushions for your joints by forming supportive connective tissue. We absolutely love collagen as a supplement, and created one called Colla-Holla in our Consult Health line. It's made from hydrolyzed collagen peptides from multiple sources (bovine, marine, chicken, egg) because each type of peptide stimulates collagen production differently; bovine can help support bone cells, marine collagen is good for skin health, and chicken/egg for joints and ligaments. Around 5,000 mg is an ideal dose. It takes time to see results from supplemental collagen, but typically after one to three months of taking it consistently, you should have fewer wrinkles, more elastic-looking skin, denser bones, and improved joint and ligament health and function.

Ashwaganda. Known as "Indian ginseng," ashwaganda has been used since 6,000 B.C. for medicinal purposes and is believed to help treat issues such as fever, anxiety, and swelling. Yet supplements made from this ingredient have only somewhat recently gained notoriety in the United States. Contemporary research has shown that it can be helpful in producing calm and reducing anxiety, producing regenerative nerve growth, and relieving pain. I've found it can improve focus and sleep, and an overall sense of well-being. Look for an ashwaganda supplement that provides 500 to 600 mg per day.

Anti-inflammatory joint supplement. As you age, you can naturally lose joint mobility and experience increased joint pain due to a decrease in lubricating fluid (synovial fluid), inflammation, and wear and tear of the smooth cartilaginous surfaces of joints. We like taking a supplement to help reduce joint-related pain by lowering inflammation. Look for one that combines anti-inflammatory ingredients like curcumin with restorative cartilage and bone-supporting calcium. These ingredients will increase joint mobility, decrease pain, and increase exercise time without pain.

I've only lost 6 pounds so far but I feel like I've lost 20. Now my stomach growls before my mind tells me I'm hungry, and my energy level and self-esteem have increased. DKFD has definitely changed my life!

—ANGELA SYES OTTO

THE DUBROW KETO FUSION DIET FOREVER

While this may be the end of the book, we hope it's just the begin-ning of a new era for you, one that's marked by achieving and main-taining your goal weight and feeling increased energy and mental clarity, all without having to endure the typical difficulties—things like excessive hunger, super-strict macronutrient rules, and boring, bland food—that are associated with diets.

We brought the DKFD to you, our readers, because we found a way to diet with science on our side. In combining fasting with selective dietary fats and strategic carbs, we discovered a way to eat that initiates fat burning (i.e., weight loss), increases mental clarity and energy, lowers inflammation, and activates your cellular anti-aging power. There's a lot here to love. If I had to pick a favorite aspect of this plan, I might say it's the flexibility around what kinds of food I can eat, while Terry is partial to the energy effects. But of course, this is kind of like trying to pick your favorite child—

This diet has completely changed my views on portion control and mental fortitude. I've seen success from this lifestyle change right out of the gate, and I look forward to seeing more.

—KEVIN EATON

they're all amazing in their own way, and combined, they're the best!

Overall, I think this diet really provides the best of everything. There aren't a lot of foods off limits (except processed stuff, which you shouldn't be eating no matter what diet plan you're following . . .). I love the fact that I can enjoy the comfort and luxury of eating richer, fattier foods and still maintain my weight, and that I feel a renewed sort of freedom around eating carbohydrates.

I remember before we started shifting to the DKFD way of eating, I used to joke that "carb" was a four-letter word for me. Like a curse word, more or less. And I think this is the case for a lot of other people, women especially. Countless times I've found myself at the gym participating in an all-female conversation where we would all confess our carb sins from the night before. But you know, this was because we were eating the types of carbs that were causing inflammation, sugar spikes, mood swings, bloat, belly fat, etc. You can almost feel this effect coming on when you eat candy, cookies, crackers, chips, and other factory carbs, as we call them.

But when we designed the Dubrow Keto Fusion Diet plan, we incorporated a way for us and for you to get carbs back into your life without any guilt. Seriously. There's no penance to be paid when you eat low-glycemic carbs. It's so liberating! "Carb" is no longer a bad four-letter word.

At the end of the day, how you eat should translate to better health, in part because this equals less need for medication or medical intervention in your life as you age. But better health also equals feeling better every single day. For me, the eating strategy and schedule of the DKFD has meant that my energy is steady, I don't get so hungry I can barely stand it (something I would experience when I wasn't getting enough fats in my diet), and my hormones feel stabilized. This last bit is huge for me. After living in hormonal hell for the last few years, it's been mind-blowing how balanced I feel eating this way; it's really become an essential part of my hormone management plan.

All this is to say, the DKFD has been a major game changer in our lives, and we hope that it will be the same for you. Thank you so much for trusting us to guide you through this journey! We always want to hear from you! Be sure to reach out to us on Instagram and join the Dubrow Keto Fusion Diet Facebook group.

Oh . . . I guess I should let Terry chime in at the end here as well. . . .

Thanks, honey. This feels a little like being second in line to sign the kids' birthday cards, but I'll take it.

I would like to personally say thank you for reading our book and for giving the metabolic science featured in the DKFD a chance to change your life. The science and strategies implemented here represent an evolution in my own personal thinking, specifically around the topic of ketogenic diets. I was always very open about the fact that I found keto to be not so smart from a medical standpoint. It's not because I doubted people could eat super-high-fat foods, protein, and essentially no carbs, and use ketones as fuel to lose weight, but I knew for certain that you couldn't do it for the rest of your life. You're never going to convince any kind of doctor that you're not supposed to have fruits and vegetables, with their cancer-preventing nutrients and antioxidants, forever. Thankfully, clinical creativity led to the development of "liberalized keto," which would provide an essential nutritional pillar to this plan, that is, the inclusion of low-glycemic carbs.

Even though the low-GI carb is sort of retro, it's been underutilized in popular diets over the last few decades. Which is why I'm so excited that with the DKFD, we have helped lead the charge to bring it back into mainstream use. Until we have personalized medicine that can bring a truly customized approach based on each individual's metabolism, eating based on a food's glycemic index—when paired with fasting and selective dietary fat intake—is what I believe to be the most powerful approach to metabolic control.

We hope that the Dubrow Keto Fusion Diet helps you achieve your weight and health goals and introduces noticeable improvements in how you feel each day. Both Heather and I have utilized the DKFD dietary strategies to great effect and we plan to keep a good thing going by continuing to eat according to 12–8–4 long-term. And we hope you will do the same!

ACKNOWLEDGMENTS

This book has been an incredible adventure! We are so grateful to our amazing support team for helping us bring this book to life.

Thank you to our kids—the Fab Four—Nick, Max, Kat, and Coco; we love you so much and we're thankful you don't roll your eyes every time we say, "So . . . we've got an idea for a new book . . ."

Thank you to everyone at HarperCollins! Lisa Sharkey, Anna Montague, Kayleigh George, Heidi Richter, Maddie Pillari, Alison Coolidge, and especially Kelly Rudolph (who knew sipping tequila with you after Sadie's bat mitzvah would result in this ?!?!). We are eternally grateful for your support in understanding the science and breakthrough technology of our fusion lifestyle plan.

Gretchen Lees: we've said it before and we will say it again— you are the hippest, coolest, smartest, funniest gal on the planet, and we are so lucky to have you in our world (and we know you and Lindsay are going to be incredible parents!).

Chef Amanda: you wow us weekly with your beautiful, DELI-CIOUS meals—and you have outdone even yourself with these un-believably yummy, easy-to-replicate dishes! Thank you for sharing your gifts!

Also, a huge thank you to Rosecleer Marie Johnson and Aziza Jade Berry, who styled the food for our photo shoot! What an art form! Speaking of photos—to our personal paparazzi, Rod Fos-ter, thank you for continuously making us look better than we deserve—LOL. Truthfully, you always capture every moment brilliantly!

Thank you to our agents, Lance Klein, Mel Berger, Ryan Mcneily, and Justin Ongert at WME, for your continued support!

Finally, our village: Natalie, Victoria, Danielle, Ina, Sue, Nora, Nicole, Rachelle, Simara, and Pete! Thank you seems insufficient, but we love you all and appreciate everything that you do!

HEATHER'S TOP SEVEN TIPS AND TRICKS FOR STAYING ON TRACK

When you're following the DKFD, you might find you experience times when sticking to the plan feels more challenging than others. I know all too well what this is like! Which is why I wanted to share with you some insider secrets to success. Some of these are ways to increase support and motivation, others are hacks to keep your head in the game . . . try out my tricks and let me know which ones helped you or share with me some of your very own!

1. Get a Support System

I've said this before, and I'll say it again—you need support to succeed on a diet. There's a reason Weight Watchers groups used to be so popular! Connecting with a community of people who have the same goal as you is super important. We'd love to be part of that community for you! I highly recommend you join our Dubrow Keto Fusion Diet Facebook group, where we chime in from time to time. You can also reach either Terry or myself on Instagram, or even call in to chat with us on our podcast if you have any questions.

2. Keep an Inspiration Board

Even if you're not a Pinterest or vision board type of person, you can benefit from simply writing down your goals and placing them where you will see them daily. I wasn't that into doing this before, but I recently put a whiteboard in my closet where I write down my goals. And I've really grown to love this pep talk and purpose reminder I've created for myself. Our twelve-year-old daughter, Katarina, has Post-its on her mirror that say, "Win a Tony award" and "Get the lead in the musical," and it's so cool to see. And she really did just get a lead in a musical, so seeing her goals each day has helped her focus on what needs to be done to help get her there.

3. Shrink Your Goal

I know this might be the opposite of what you usually hear, which is to go big or go home, or whatever cheesy, sports-based slogan you might encounter around the topic of goal setting. But sometimes a big goal can feel like an enormous mountain you have to climb, making even those first few steps intimidating. Try shrinking the mountain to make getting going a little easier for you.

Like we mentioned in the beginning of the book, create an initial goal to lose just 5 percent of your weight. A 5 percent weight loss will provide enormous benefits, shrinking the visceral fat that accumulates around your organs, dropping just enough of the baggage you're carrying around to help you feel less sluggish and more motivated to keep going.

You'll be surprised—minimizing your goal can maximize your results in the long run.

4. Game the System

This tip pertains specifically to exercise. I sometimes find that exercise can be boring, and that's the case even though I love doing it quite a bit. To help keep myself in the game, I start to literally play games in my head. For example, when I do any kind of machine-based cardio workout and I'm on the treadmill or rower, I will try to look at the numbers and identify patterns or cut the time down into small segments—like, "C'mon, Heather—just get through the next 30 seconds, and then the next, and then the next . . . ," and then suddenly you're done! Sometimes you literally have to trick your brain to get your body through a workout.

5. Honor the Experience of Eating

Some people eat to live and some live to eat. If you're the former type of person, you probably can identify with the idea of food being fuel. People who live to eat, on the other hand, find the idea of food being fuel utterly depressing—they want eating to be fun, enjoyable, even provide an *experience*.

If you're the type of person who lives to eat, you might have had a hard time following any kind of eating plan in the past— because you want the whole enchilada, so to speak. A nice atmosphere, cute plates, nice-looking food, utensils in order, and so on. And you might have become convinced that the only place you can have this experience is at a restaurant. But this isn't true! You can create it all for yourself at home.

I encourage you, no matter what type of eater you are, to create the best experience for yourself when you're following this plan and make beautiful meals for yourself out of your own kitchen. Don't eat your meals while leaning over the counter or off a paper plate— build your plate of food, use a place mat, and sit down to a nice meal. You can do this whether you're with your family or significant other, or on your own—the experience of eating will be enriched either way. And try staying off social media and keeping the TV off. Give yourself the chance to enjoy undistracted eating. See how getting better connected to your food makes you feel. I bet you'll feel it's more enjoyable, and you'll experience greater appetite satisfaction.

Then, once you're done with your meal and cleanup, get out of the kitchen! If you hang out in the kitchen, you'll find something to keep munching on even if you're not hungry.

You can control your environment even when you're traveling, too. Everyone knows airplane food is the worst. Pack up a nice meal for yourself and toss it in your tote, purse, or backpack. And include snacks like beef jerky, roasted nuts, or even deviled eggs. This way, when you get through security and you're already hungry, you'll have something to nosh on before your flight.

6. Create an End-of-Meal Ritual

I recommend closing the book on eating for the day with some sort of ritual. Have a cup of tea, pop a mint in your mouth, brush your teeth, or do something else similar. If you try to do this most nights, it will become a signal that it's time to let your digestion wind down into fasting for the next 12 hours.

7. Losing Motivation? Treat Yourself with a Nonfood Reward

Sometimes all you need is a little treat to restore your interest and investment in an endeavor. If you've been sticking to the DKFD diligently and you are making progress, create a reward point for yourself. If you've reached your 5-percent weight loss goal, get a massage or go get a mani-pedi at the fancy spa place that you save for special occasions. Or go get yourself a new workout bra (or shorts or shirt, if you're a guy). . . . Do something that makes you feel good!

SELECTED REFERENCES

In writing this book, we referenced the following sources:

Introduction

Dateline. "The Ketogenic Diet." Aired October 26, 1994, on NBC.

Magkos, Faidon, Gemma Fraterrigo, Jun Yoshino, Courtney Luecking, Kyleigh Kirbach, Shannon C. Kelly, Lisa De Las Fuentes, et al. "Effects of Moderate and Subsequent Progressive Weight Loss on Metabolic Function and Adipose Tissue Biology in Humans with Obesity." *Cell Metabolism* 23, no. 4 (2016): 591–601. https://doi.org/10.1016/j.cmet.2016.02.005.

Chapter 1

Bailey, Melissa. "Sugar Industry Secretly Paid for Favorable Harvard Research." STAT. September 12, 2016. https://www.statnews.com/2016/09/12/sugar-industry-harvard-research/.

Buyken, Anette E., Janina Goletzke, Gesa Joslowski, Anna Felbick, Guo Cheng, Christian Herder, and Jennie C. Brand-Miller. "Association Between Carbohydrate Quality and Inflammatory Markers: Systematic Review of Observational and Interventional Studies." *American Journal of Clinical Nutrition* 99, no. 4 (2014): 813–33. https://doi.org/10.3945/ajcn.113.074252.

Feinman, Richard D., and Eugene J. Fine. "'A Calorie Is a Calorie' Violates the Second Law of Thermodynamics." *Nutrition Journal* 3, no. 9 (2004). https://doi.org/10.1186/1475-2891-3-9.

Harper, Hugo, and Michael Hallsworth. *Counting Calories: How Under-Reporting Can Explain the Apparent Fall in Calorie Intake*. London: The Behavioral Insights Team, 2016. https://www.bi.team/wp-content/uploads/2016/08/16-07-12-Counting-Calories-Final.pdf.

Kowalski, Greg M., Steven Hamley, Ahrathy Selathurai, Joachim Kloehn, David P. De Souza, Sean O'Callaghan, Brunda Nijagal, Dedreia L. Tull, Malcolm J. Mcconville, and Clinton R. Bruce. "Reversing Diet-Induced Metabolic Dysregulation by Diet Switching Leads to Altered Hepatic De Novo Lipogenesis and Glycerolipid Synthesis." *Scientific Reports* 6, no. 1 (2016). https://doi.org/10.1038/srep27541.

La Berge, Ann F. "How the Ideology of Low Fat Conquered America." *Journal of the History of Medicine and Allied Sciences* 63, no. 2 (2008): 139–77. https://doi.org/10.1093/jhmas/jrn001.

McGandy, Robert B., D. M. Hegsted, and F. J. Stare. "Dietary Fats, Carbohydrates and Atherosclerotic Vascular Disease." *New England Journal of Medicine* 277, no. 4 (1967): 186–92. https://doi.org/10.1056/nejm196707272770405.

Mozaffarian, Dariush, and David S. Ludwig. "The 2015 US Dietary Guidelines: Lifting the Ban on Total Dietary Fat." *Journal of the American Medical Association* 313, no. 24 (2015): 2421–22. https://doi.org/10.1001/jama.2015.5941.

Pfeifer, Heidi H., and Elizabeth A. Thiele. "Low-Glycemic-Index Treatment: A Liberalized Ketogenic Diet for Treatment of Intractable Epilepsy." *Neurology* 65, no. 11 (December 2005): 1810–12. https://doi.org/10.1212/01.wnl.0000187071.24292.9e.

Qi, Xin, and Richard F. Tester. "The 'Epileptic Diet'-Ketogenic and/or Slow Release of Glucose Intervention: A Review." *Clinical Nutrition* 19 (2019): 30253–55.

Singleton, J. Robinson, A. Gordon Smith, and Robin L. Marcus. "Exercise as Therapy for Diabetic and Prediabetic Neuropathy." *Current Diabetes Reports* 15, no. 12 (2015). https://doi.org/10.1007/s11892-015-0682–6.

"Trends in Adult Body-Mass Index in 200 Countries from 1975 to 2014: A Pooled Analysis of 1698 Population-Based Measurement Studies with 19.2 Million Participants." *Lancet* 387, no. 10026 (2016): 1377–96. https://doi.org/10.1016/s0140-6736(16)30054-x.

World Health Organization. "Obesity and Overweight." World Health Organization Fact Sheet. February 16, 2018. https://www.who.int/news-room/fact-sheets/detail/obesity-and-overweight.

Yancy, William S., Jr., Maren K. Olsen, John R. Guyton, Ronna P. Bakst, and Eric C. Westman. "A Low-Carbohydrate, Ketogenic Diet versus a Low-Fat Diet to Treat Obesity and Hyperlipidemia: A Randomized, Controlled Trial." *Annals of Internal Medicine* 140, no. 10 (2004):769–77. https://doi.org/10.7326/0003-4819-140-10-200405180-00006.

Yancy, William S., Jr., Marjorie Foy, Allison M. Chalecki, Mary C. Vernon, and Eric C. Westman. "A Low-Carbohydrate, Ketogenic Diet to Treat Type 2 Diabetes." *Nutrition & Metabolism* 2, no. 34 (2005). https://doi.org/10.1186/1743-7075-2-34.

Chapter 3

Bansal, Devika G. "How Ketogenic Diets Curb Inflammation in the Brain." University of California, San Francisco, News. September 27, 2019. https://www.ucsf.edu/news/2017/09/408366/how-ketogenic-diets-curb-inflammation-brain.

Browning, Jeffrey D., Jeannie Baxter, Santhosh Satapati, and Shawn C. Burgess. "The Effect of Short-Term Fasting on Liver and Skeletal Muscle Lipid, Glucose, and Energy Metabolism in Healthy Women and Men." *Journal of Lipid Research* 53, no. 3 (March 2011): 577–86. https://doi.org/10.1194/jlr.p020867.

Dehghan, Mahshid, Andrew Mente, Xiaohe Zhang, Sumathi Swaminathan, Wei Li, Viswanathan Mohan, Romaina Iqbal, et al. "Associations of Fats and Carbohydrate Intake with Cardiovascular Disease and Mortality in 18 Countries from Five Continents (PURE): A Prospective Cohort Study." *Lancet* 390, no. 10107 (2017): 2050–62. https://doi.org/10.1016/S0140-6736(17)32252-3.

Fromentin, Claire, Daniel Tomé, Françoise Nau, Laurent Flet, Catherine Luengo, Dalila Azzout-Marniche, Pascal Sanders, Gilles Fromentin, and Claire Gaudichon. "Dietary Proteins Contribute Little to Glucose Production, Even Under Optimal Gluconeogenic Conditions in Healthy Humans." *Diabetes* 62, no. 5 (2013): 1435–42. https://doi.org/10.2337/db12-1208.

Furmli, Suleiman, Rami Elmasry, Megan Ramos, and Jason Fung. "Therapeutic Use of Intermittent Fasting for People with Type 2 Diabetes as an Alternative to Insulin." *BMJ Case Reports* (September 2018). https://doi.org/10.1136/bcr-2017-221854.

Goodpaster, Bret H., and Lauren M. Sparks. "Metabolic Flexibility in Health and Disease." *Cell Metabolism* 25, no. 5 (2017): 1027–36. https://doi.org/10.1016/j.cmet.2017.04.015.

Harcombe, Zoë, Julien S. Baker, Stephen Mark Cooper, Bruce Davies, Nicholas Sculthorpe, James J. Dinicolantonio, and Fergal Grace. "Evidence from Randomised Controlled Trials Did Not Support the Introduction of Dietary Fat Guidelines in 1977 and 1983: A Systematic Review and Meta-Analysis." *Open Heart* 2, no. 1 (2015). https://doi.org/10.1136/openhrt-2014-000196.

Ivanova, Ekaterina A., Veronika A. Myasoedova, Alexandra A. Melnichenko, Andrey V. Grechko, and Alexander N. Orekhov. "Small Dense Low-Density Lipoprotein as Biomarker for Atherosclerotic Diseases." *Oxidative Medicine and Cellular Longevity* 2017 (2017): 1–10. https://doi.org/10.1155/2017/1273042.

Izuta, Yusuke, Toshihiro Imada, Ryuji Hisamura, Erina Oonishi, Shigeru Nakamura, Emi Inagaki, Masataka Ito, Tomoyoshi Soga, and Kazuo Tsubota. "Ketone Body 3-Hydroxybutyrate Mimics Calorie Restriction via the Nrf2 Activator, Fumarate, in the Retina." *Aging Cell* 17, no. 1 (2017). https://doi.org/10.1111/acel.12699.

Mattson, Mark P., and Ruiqian Wan. "Beneficial Effects of Intermittent Fasting and Caloric Restriction on the Cardiovascular and Cerebrovascular Systems." *Journal of Nutritional Biochemistry* 16, no. 3 (2005): 129–37. https://doi.org/10.1016/j.jnutbio.2004.12.007.

Mumme, Karen, and Welma Stonehouse. "Effects of Medium-Chain Triglycerides on Weight Loss and Body Composition: A Meta-Analysis of Randomized Controlled Trials." *Journal of the Academy of Nutrition and Dietetics* 115, no. 2 (2015): 249–63. https://doi.org/10.1016/j.jand.2014.10.022.

Niramitmahapanya, Sathit, Susan S. Harris, and Bess Dawson-Hughes. "Type of Dietary Fat Is Associated with the 25-Hydroxyvitamin D3 Increment in Response to Vitamin D Supplementation." *Journal of Clinical Endocrinology & Metabolism* 96, no. 10 (2011): 3170–74. https://doi.org/10.1210/jc.2011-1518.

Ormazabal, Valeska, Soumyalekshmi Nair, Omar Elfeky, Claudio Aguayo, Carlos Salomon, and Felipe A. Zuñiga. "Association Between Insulin Resistance and the Development of Cardiovascular Disease." *Cardiovascular Diabetology* 17, no. 1 (2018). https://doi.org/10.1186/s12933-018-0762-4.

Paoli, Antonio, Gerardo Bosco, Enrico M. Camporesi, and Devanand Mangar. "Ketosis, Ketogenic Diet and Food Intake Control: A Complex Relationship." *Frontiers in Psychology* 6, no. 27 (2015). https://doi.org/10.3389/fpsyg.2015.00027.

Siri-Tarino, Patty W., Qi Sun, Frank B. Hu, and Ronald M. Krauss. "Meta-Analysis of Prospective Cohort Studies Evaluating the Association of Saturated Fat with Cardiovascular Disease." *American Journal of Clinical Nutrition* 91, no. 3 (2010): 535–46. https://doi.org/10.3945/ajcn.2009.27725.

Uddin, Md. Sahab, Anna Stachowiak, Abdullah Al Mamun, Nikolay T. Tzvetkov, Shinya Takeda, Atanas G. Atanasov, Leandro B. Bergantin, Mohamed M. Abdel-Daim, and Adrian M. Stankiewicz. "Autophagy and Alzheimer's Disease: From Molecular Mechanisms to Therapeutic Implications." *Frontiers in Aging Neuroscience* 10 (2018). https://doi.org/10.3389/fnagi.2018.00004.

Wang, Yang, Peter Dellatore, Veronique Douard, Ling Qin, Malcolm Watford, Ronaldo P. Ferraris, Tiao Lin, and Sue A. Shapses. "High Fat Diet Enriched with Saturated, but Not Monounsaturated Fatty Acids Adversely Affects Femur, and Both Diets Increase Calcium Absorption in Older Female Mice." *Nutrition Research* 36, no. 7 (2016): 742–50. https://doi.org/10.1016/j.nutres.2016.03.002.

Yesikar, Veena, Rajendra Kumar Mahore, Sanjay Dixit, Geeta Shivram, Shailesh Rai, Sachin Parmar, and Surendra Mahore. "An Observational Study to Assess the Physical, Social, Psychological and Spiritual Aspects of Fasting." *IOSR Journal of Dental and Medical Sciences* 14, no. 3 (2015): 25–30.

Youm, Yun-Hee, Kim Y. Nguyen, Ryan W. Grant, Emily L. Goldberg, Monica Bodogai, Dongin Kim, Dominic Dagostino, et al. "The Ketone Metabolite ß-Hydroxybutyrate Blocks NLRP3 Inflammasome–Mediated Inflammatory Disease." *Nature Medicine* 21, no. 3 (2015): 263–69. https://doi.org/10.1038/nm.3804.

Chapter 4

Anderson, James W., Kim M. Randles, Cyril W. C. Kendall, and David J. A. Jenkins. "Carbohydrate and Fiber Recommendations for Individuals with Diabetes: A Quantitative Assessment and Meta-Analysis of the Evidence." *Journal of the American College of Nutrition* 23, no. 1 (2004): 5–17. https://doi.org/10.1080/07315724.2004.10719338.

Beulens, Joline W. J., Leonie M. de Bruijne, Ronald P. Stolk, Petra H. M. Peeters, Michiel L. Bots, Diederick E. Grobbee, and Yvonne T. van der Schouw. "High Dietary Glycemic Load and Glycemic Index Increase Risk of Cardiovascular Disease Among Middle-Aged Women: A Population-Based Follow-Up Study." *Journal of the American College of Cardiology* 50, no. 1 (2007): 14–21. https://doi .org/10.1016/j.jacc.2007.02.068.

Björntorp, P. "The Regulation of Adipose Tissue Distribution in Humans." *International Journal of Obesity and Related Metabolic Disorders: Journal of the International Association for the Study of Obesity* 20, no. 4 (1996): 291–302.

Chavarro, J. E., J. W. Rich-Edwards, B. A. Rosner, and W. C. Willett. "A Prospective Study of Dietary Carbohydrate Quantity and Quality in Relation to Risk of Ovulatory Infertility." *European Journal of Clinical Nutrition* 63, no. 1 (2009): 78–86. https://doi.org/10.1038/sj.ejcn.1602904.

Chiu, C. J., L. D. Hubbard, J. Armstrong, G. Rogers, P. F. Jacques, L. T. Chylack, S. E. Hankinson, W. C. Willett, and A. Taylor. "Dietary Glycemic Index and Carbohydrate in Relation to Early Age-Related Macular Degeneration." *American Journal of Ophthalmology* 142, no. 3 (2006): 535–36. https://doi.org/10.1016 /j.ajo.2006.07.011.

De Munter, Jeroen S. L., Frank B. Hu, Donna Spiegelman, Mary Franz, and Rob M. van Dam. "Whole Grain, Bran, and Germ Intake and Risk of Type 2 Diabetes: A Prospective Cohort Study and Systematic Review." *PLoS Medicine* 4, no. 8 (2007). https://doi.org/10.1371/journal.pmed.0040261.

Ebbeling, Cara B., Michael M. Leidig, Henry A. Feldman, Margaret M. Lovesky, and David S. Ludwig. "Effects of a Low–Glycemic Load vs Low-Fat Diet in Obese Young Adults." *Journal of the American Medical Association* 297, no. 19 (2007): 2092. https://doi.org/10.1001/jama.297.19.2092.

Harcombe, Zoë, Julien S. Baker, Stephen Mark Cooper, Bruce Davies, Nicholas Sculthorpe, James J. DiNicolantonio, and Fergal Grace. "Evidence from Randomised Controlled Trials Did Not Support the Introduction of Dietary Fat Guidelines in 1977 and 1983: A Systematic Review and Meta-Analysis." *Open Heart* 2, no. 1 (2015). https://doi.org/10.1136/openhrt-2014-000196.

Higginbotham, Susan, Zuo-Feng Zhang, I-Min Lee, Nancy R. Cook, Edward Giovannucci, Julie E. Buring, and Simin Liu. "Dietary Glycemic Load and Risk of Colorectal Cancer in the Women's Health Study." *Journal of the National Cancer Institute* 96, no. 3 (2004): 229–33. https://doi.org/10.1093/jnci/djh020.

Jovanovski, Elena, Andreea Zurbau, and Vladimir Vuksan. "Carbohydrates and Endothelial Function: Is a Low-Carbohydrate Diet or a Low-Glycemic Index Diet Favourable for Vascular Health?" *Clinical Nutrition Research* 4, no. 2 (2015): 69–75. https://doi.org/10.7762/cnr.2015.4.2.69.

Livesey, Geoffrey, Richard Taylor, Helen F. Livesey, Anette E. Buyken, David J. A. Jenkins, Livia S. A. Augustin, John L. Sievenpiper, et al. "Dietary Glycemic Index and Load and the Risk of Type 2 Diabetes: A Systematic Review and Updated

Meta-Analyses of Prospective Cohort Studies." *Nutrients* 11, no. 6 (2019): 1280. https://doi.org/10.3390/nu11061280.

Ludwig, David S., Joseph A. Majzoub, Ahmad Al-Zahrani, Gerard E. Dallal, Isaac Blanco, and Susan B. Roberts. "High Glycemic Index Foods, Overeating, and Obesity." *Pediatrics* 103, no. 3 (1999). https://doi.org/10.1542/peds.103.3.e26.

Maki, Kevin C., Tia M. Rains, Valerie N. Kaden, Kathleen R. Raneri, and Michael H. Davidson. "Effects of a Reduced-Glycemic-Load Diet on Body Weight, Body Composition, and Cardiovascular Disease Risk Markers in Overweight and Obese Adults." *American Journal of Clinical Nutrition* 85, no. 3 (2007): 724–34. https://doi.org/10.1093/ajcn/85.3.724.

Sofer, Sigal, Abraham Eliraz, Sara Kaplan, Hillary Voet, Gershon Fink, Tzadok Kima, and Zecharia Madar. "Greater Weight Loss and Hormonal Changes After 6 Months Diet with Carbohydrates Eaten Mostly at Dinner." *Obesity* 19, no. 10 (2011): 2006–14. https://doi.org/10.1038/oby.2011.48.

Wolever, Thomas M. S., David J. A. Jenkins, Anthony M. Ocana, Venketeshwer A. Rao, and Gregory R. Collier. "Second-Meal Effect: Low-Glycemic-Index Foods Eaten at Dinner Improve Subsequent Breakfast Glycemic Response." *American Journal of Clinical Nutrition* 48, no. 4 (1988): 1041–47. https://doi.org/10.1093/ajcn/48.4.1041.

Chapter 5

American Chemical Society. "New Low-Calorie Rice Could Help Cut Rising Obesity Rates." News release. March 23, 2015. https://www.acs.org/content/acs/en/pressroom/newsreleases/2015/march/new-low-calorie-rice-could-help-cut-rising-obesity-rates.html.

Keyes, Katherine M., Esteban Calvo, Katherine A. Ornstein, Caroline Rutherford, Matthew P. Fox, Ursula M. Staudinger, and Linda P. Fried. "Alcohol Consumption in Later Life and Mortality in the United States: Results from 9 Waves of the Health and Retirement Study." *Alcoholism: Clinical and Experimental Research* 43, no. 8 (2019): 1734–46. https://doi.org/10.1111/acer.14125.

Sonia, Steffi, Fiastuti Witjaksono, and Rahmawati Ridwan. "Effect of Cooling of Cooked White Rice on Resistant Starch Content and Glycemic Response." *Asia Pacific Journal of Clinical Nutrition* 24, no. 4 (2015): 620–25. https://doi.org/10.6133/apjcn.2015.24.4.13.

Chapter 7

Mayo Clinic Staff. "Exercise: 7 Benefits of Regular Physical Activity." Healthy Lifestyle: Fitness. May 11, 2019. https://www.mayoclinic.org/healthy-lifestyle/fitness/in-depth/exercise/art-20048389.

Chiu, Chung-Jung, Larry D. Hubbard, Jane Armstrong, Gail Rogers, Paul F. Jacques, Leo T. Chylack, Jr., Susan E. Hankinson, Walter C. Willett, and Allen Taylor. "Dietary Glycemic Index and Carbohydrate in Relation to Early Age-Related Macular Degeneration." *American Journal of Clinical Nutrition* 83, no. 4 (2006): 880–86. https://doi.org/10.1093/ajcn/83.4.880.

Singh, Narendra, Mohit Bhalla, Prashanti de Jager, and Marilena Gilca. "An Overview on Ashwagandha: A Rasayana (Rejuvenator) of Ayurveda." *African Journal of Traditional, Complementary and Alternative Medicines* 8, no. S5 (2011): 208–13. https://doi.org/10.4314/ajtcam.v8i5S.9.

INDEX

*Index entries in **bold** indicate recipe titles.*

ABOUT THE AUTHORS

HEATHER DUBROW is an actress, television personality, author, and the host of the top-rated podcast *Heather Dubrow's World*. Heather and her husband, Dr. Terry Dubrow, have the #1-selling skin care and supplement line, Consult Beaute & Health, which is sold exclusively on the ShopHQ shopping channel. Heather and Terry live in California with their four children.

On Instagram and Twitter: @heatherdubrow

On Facebook: @heatherdubrowofficial

Website: heatherdubrow.com

DR. TERRY DUBROW obtained degrees in the medical sciences from Yale University in 1980 and the UCLA School of Medicine in 1986. He is certified by the American Board of Plastic Surgery and is also a certified expert for the Medical Board of California. Dr. Dubrow has been showcased as the surgical expert on several television shows, including FOX's *The Swan* and E!'s *Bridalplasty*, and since 2013, he has been the star of E!'s hit show *Botched*. He and his wife, Heather, live in California with their four children.

On Instagram, Twitter, and Facebook: @drdubrow

Website: drdubrow.com